TORONTO

BOSTON & CAMBRIDGE

BROOKLYN

WASHINGTON, D.C.

EVOLVING VEGAN

EVOLVING VEGAN

DELICIOUSLY DIVERSE RECIPES FROM NORTH AMERICA'S BEST PLANT-BASED EATERIES— FOR ANYONE WHO LOVES FOOD

MENA MASSOUD

TILLER PRESS

NEW YORK   LONDON   TORONTO   SYDNEY   NEW DELHI

TILLER PRESS

An Imprint of Simon & Schuster, Inc.
1230 Avenue of the Americas
New York, NY 10020

First Tiller Press hardcover edition September 2020

TILLER PRESS and colophon are trademarks of Simon & Schuster, Inc.

For information about special discounts for bulk purchases,
please contact Simon & Schuster Special Sales at 1-866-506-1949
or business@simonandschuster.com.

The Simon & Schuster Speakers Bureau can bring authors to your
live event. For more information or to book an event, contact the
Simon & Schuster Speakers Bureau at 1-866-248-3049 or visit
our website at www.simonspeakers.com.

Interior design by Matt Ryan
Photography by Andrew Rowley
Author photo on page 192 by Alexi Lubomirski

Manufactured in the United States of America

10 9 8 7 6 5 4 3 2 1

Library of Congress Cataloging-in-Publication Data

Names: Massoud, Mena, author.
Title: Evolving vegan : deliciously diverse recipes from North America's
best plant-based eateries-for anyone who loves food / Mena Massoud.
Identifiers: LCCN 2020010320 (print) | LCCN 2020010321 (ebook) | ISBN
9781982144562 (hardcover) | ISBN 9781982144579 (ebook)
Subjects: LCSH: Vegan cooking—North America. | LCGFT: Cookbooks.
Classification: LCC TX837 .M23667 2020 (print) | LCC TX837 (ebook) | DDC
641.5/6362—dc23
LC record available at https://lccn.loc.gov/2020010320
LC ebook record available at https://lccn.loc.gov/2020010321

ISBN 978-1-9821-4456-2
ISBN 978-1-9821-4457-9 (ebook)

DEDICATED TO MY BEAUTIFUL MOM, GORGIT, WHO SPARKED MY PASSION FOR FOOD, COOKING, AND THE ENTERTAINMENT OF OTHERS. LOVE YOU, MA.

CONTE

A FEW YEARS AGO, WHEN I FIRST ADOPTED A PLANT-BASED LIFESTYLE, I WAS QUITE CONFIDENT THAT VEGAN LIVING WAS GOING TO TAKE OVER THE WORLD VERY RAPIDLY. FIVE YEARS LATER, IT'S CLEAR TO ME THAT WHILE IT MAY NOT BE HAPPENING AS QUICKLY AS I WANT IT TO, THE WORLD IS CERTAINLY EVOLVING VEGAN.

Most people are not completely vegan, committing themselves to a lifestyle void of all animal products, ocean life, animal by-products like honey, and materials made from animals, like leather and fur. But people are aware of the impact all those things have on our planet, and more people are trying to limit their consumption of animal products. And that is a victory in itself. In the last year alone, some of the biggest fast-food chains in the world have introduced numerous plant-based options. The reason these big conglomerates have invested millions into plant-based food is not necessarily that they see the number of hard-core vegans increasing; it's because they are noticing a shift in how meat-eaters are consuming food—most people truly are evolving vegan.

So while the majority of people in America still consider themselves "meat-eaters," they are beginning to consume considerably less animal products and more plant-based foods. Whether that's by switching to plant-based milks for their coffee or implementing Meatless Monday, there's a tectonic shift happening in what people are consuming and how they are consuming it. Humans are starting to take responsibility for the major changes happening to our planet and their own health. And you don't need to become a militant vegan to make a difference.

Even when it comes to my personal lifestyle, I can't call myself 100% vegan. That's the whole reason I started Evolving Vegan, the company. Why? Because like with any other label, group, or cult, there are very specific rules to which you have to adhere to be able to label yourself "vegan." And to be frank (who the hell is Frank, anyway?) I don't like locking myself in chains made up of a set of specific rules just because a group of people got together one day and decided what it takes to qualify as a "vegan," deeming any person outside those stipulations an outsider or unworthy. So here's what I say:

Try your hardest to cut down your intake of animal products, do your part to reduce your environmental footprint, and start taking pride in what you put into your body, because you know it's better for your health. That's what it means to be evolving vegan, and everyone is welcome.

The majority of the friends I cook for or take out to plant-based restaurants tell me the same thing: "If I could eat vegan food like this all the time, I would be vegan." And at first, the Al Pacino part of my brain wants to look them intensely in the eyes, peering down into their soul to the very being of who they are, strangle them, and yell very loudly, "YOU'RE IN THE DARK HERE! YOU UNDERSTAND?! YOU'RE IN THE DARK!" That's a slight variation on what Pacino actually says in *Scent of a Woman*, but you get my point. After a moment of reason, however, I explain to my friends that while it's not as easy and accessible, yes, they *can* eat like this every day, and they don't have to become a raw, organic, only-comes-from-trees herbivore overnight. They can start off slow, committing to eating plant-based two days a week, which eventually evolves into only eating meat twice a week, which turns into only eating it when they have no other choice (and to be honest, I think you always have a choice).

THE ANIMAL DISCUSSION

Many vegans switched to a plant-based lifestyle because of their love and compassion for animals. I did it because of my love for the earth and for my health. Let's be real here. Yes, it is absolutely horrendous how animals are farmed to accommodate our eating habits. And anyone who even remotely loves animals should really think twice about the hypocrisy they are living. But you have to remember that for generations before factory farms existed, and still to this day, tribes and groups of humans all over the world have hunted with their fellow animal counterparts. In Mongolia, hunters track game with eagles as their partners, and the eagles always get to eat first (usually the heart or liver of their prey). It's primal. It's natural. It's part of the circle of life. But the point is, humans have evolved as a species to the point where we don't *have to* eat that way anymore. We don't have to kill other animals in order to survive and prosper. We don't have to farm and enslave any kind of animal at the expense of our planet's well-being. Let me be clear: I care about the animals, I really do. But without the planet, without Mother Nature, there are no animals, there is no vegetation, and there is no us. And the most important thing you can do to reduce your environmental impact is to change the way you eat. (Do that first, and then buy an electric vehicle and line your roof with solar panels and you're pretty much Gandhi.) Not only will you be doing your part to prolong the life of our beautiful planet, but you'll start to appreciate all living life the same—not only the cute dogs that you get to pet in your neighborhood. Just because you don't see the animals you end up consuming doesn't mean they don't have the same spirit and desire to live as the animals we see day to day. Eat more plants and less meat, and you'll be helping to save our planet and doing wonders for your health at the same time.

And no, I won't get into the specifics of that or try to debunk the idea that some people's "blood types" need meat, because that's not what this book is about.

WHAT I ATE GROWING UP

My parents were very traditional, so, as you can imagine, I grew up speaking Arabic, studying my ass off to become a doctor, and eating pretty much every part of every animal you can consume: kidney, liver, heart, intestine, stomach lining, hooves, fish guts (not caviar—who has money for that?). I even scored me some tongue—of a cow, that is. I mean, I grew up eating food so crazy-sounding that if I had told anyone at school, they would have run the other way so fast, I wouldn't have had the time to repeat my name to them fifteen times.

If you've ever eaten any of these, you are automatically part of the Massoud club:

- Rice and pita bread (so far so good), soaked in beef broth and served with cow hooves
- Medley of kidney, liver, and heart, panfried with butter, onion, tons of garlic, and jalapeños, served with warm pita bread
- Cow intestine stuffed with Mediterranean rice

Needless to say, I have tried a wider variety of foods than many people on Earth, simply because of my heritage. And because of that, I think I developed quite a good palate. When I transitioned to a plant-based diet, I did crave a lot of that food, but over time, your body adjusts, and I actually feel like I cleansed my palate in a lot of ways. All of a sudden, vegetables had a lot more flavor, legumes started to feel hearty and satisfying, and I felt so much lighter! It's very similar to what happens when you cut out processed simple sugars from your diet, and after a while, fruits start to taste sweeter than they ever have before.

My love for cooking was embedded in me at a young age because my mom cooked for us every night of the week, sometimes two or three times on a Saturday or Sunday, and on holidays, well, just forget about it—we could have fed our whole neighborhood. Food has always been a passion of mine, and I have enjoyed navigating this world of plant-based cuisine more than I ever imagined I would.

THE VEGAN VISIONARIES

This book is about the incredible stories of chefs and restaurateurs around North America. Visionaries who were ahead of the curve, who took the chance when people told them there was no way an establishment that doesn't serve meat could survive. Plant-based eaters who are doing their part and making vegan food accessible—changing exactly what nonvegans always complain about ("If I could eat vegan food like this all the time, I would be vegan"). These are my favorite places to eat in North America, so when you're traveling and seeing what cities our great Earth, our great species has created, you can do your part and help protect the planet by visiting these kick-ass restaurants. Not only that, but I've gone one step further and included a recipe from or inspired by each of these establishments, so the next time you want to complain about "not knowing what to cook that's plant-based," you'll have a plethora of options. There are plenty of books, documentaries, articles, journals, and resources that can help with debunking your doubts, insecurities, and irrational arguments. And because I'm such a nice guy, I have included a list of these top educational resources at the end of this book. So, in the spirit of Guy Fieri, here are my top plant-based establishments around North America, and once again, this . . . is *Evolving Vegan*.

THE BOOK

One of the reasons I created this book was to tear down the stereotype of the typical "cookbook." Most people who aren't experts in culinary literature often associate cookbooks with female celebrities (chefs or otherwise) and a bunch of pretty photos of them and their food in heavenly harmony with their spotless kitchens, which look like they were designed for the rich and famous. And you know what? Everybody needs a little bit of Martha once in a while, but she definitely doesn't represent the majority of cooks or households in America.

Food is fun and cooking is accessible. If there's anything the late Anthony Bourdain taught us, it's that gastronomy is never one thing. It cannot be defined by rules or stipulations made up by a group of people, and neither should your favorite cookbook. Cooking and enjoying food with one another is a universal truth, one that brings people together and bonds them in that very tradition. It's what separates us from many other species on Earth. So I traveled North America, checking out the best plant-based establishments in our great cities and compiling recipes inspired by those incredible bars, restaurants, dives, and cafés. I created this book so that you could follow my journey and re-create some of these delicious flavors at home. You don't have to look like Martha or have her kitchen to cook these recipes, and you might not even want to follow any of these recipes exactly as written. Maybe you'll just be inspired by the photos we captured, the cities we visited, and the stories we gathered.

And just to be clear, here are all the different categories of recipes in the book:

RECIPES FROM A RESTAURANT: These restaurants were kind enough to give us the (almost) identical recipes they use in their actual kitchens. We may have simplified a sauce so you don't have to go out and buy thirty-seven ingredients, but the recipe is pretty much how you'd find it at the restaurant.

RECIPES INSPIRED BY A RESTAURANT: These are recipes that I came up with after I visited a restaurant and tried their version of a dish. So while the photo we captured is from our actual tour, the recipe has my little twist on it.

RECIPES FROM MY HOME KITCHEN: These are my go-to recipes, the ones I cook on a regular basis. I love having a repertoire from which I can cook every night, even if I'm practicing juggling, rehearsing a dance number, and singing all at the same time. And I hope they become your favorites, too.

RECIPES FROM MAMMA'S KITCHEN: For years I've been stressing out about how I can preserve my mom's recipes for future generations. Then I thought, what better way to keep my mom's recipes alive than in a cookbook? These are my favorite recipes in the whole book. Thank you, Ma!

PANTRY ESSENTIALS

Just a few things to keep in mind as you make these recipes:

WHEN "NEUTRAL OIL" is specified, feel free to use any of the following: avocado, sunflower, safflower, or grapeseed oil. You can also substitute any one of these for the other.

ALSO FEEL FREE TO USE GLUTEN-FREE FLOUR, bread, or bread crumbs in any of these recipes that call for the conventional type. Please note that the gluten-free flour used in this cookbook includes xanthan gum.

USE YOUR FAVORITE TYPE OF NONDAIRY MILK in these recipes, be it almond, oat, cashew, or otherwise. Keep in mind, different milks will give you different results—don't be afraid to experiment!

ALL NUT BUTTERS should be all natural and stirred before using.

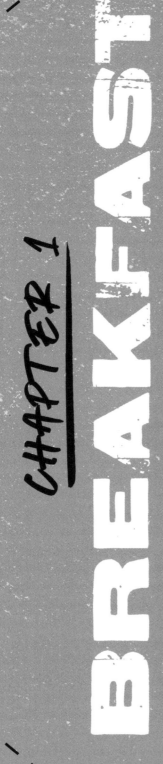

CHAPTER 1
BREAKFAST

Featuring recipes from or inspired by:

BODHI BOWL
LOS ANGELES, CALIFORNIA

BUTCHER'S DAUGHTER
LOS ANGELES, CALIFORNIA

CHICKPEA
VANCOUVER, CANADA

HEIRLOOM
VANCOUVER, CANADA

LITTLE CHOC APOTHECARY
BROOKLYN, NEW YORK

MY HOME KITCHEN

OFF THE GRIDDLE
PORTLAND, OREGON

TRILOGY SANCTUARY
SAN DIEGO, CALIFORNIA

STICKY FINGERS SWEETS & EATS
WASHINGTON, DC

SWEET HART KITCHEN
TORONTO, CANADA

VEGGIE GALAXY
CAMBRIDGE, MASSACHUSETTS

AÇAI BOWL

MAKES ABOUT 6 CUPS GRANOLA

Açai has blown up over the past few years. We live in an age of social media when, once in a while, even fruits and vegetables can go viral. So why is everyone bananas about açai? (See what I did there, a pun with two different fruits?) Research does show that açai berry pulp is richer in antioxidants than other berries, but claims of its antiaging and weight-loss properties have not been backed up with any substantial evidence. My opinion is that it's mostly just a trend. The other downside is that you almost never see fresh açai berries in stores. It's most often sold as a frozen puree, but lucky for us, that's exactly what we need in this recipe! I love the açai bowl for its subtle flavor and versatility, but most shops will charge anywhere from $10 to $15 for one serving, so I wanted to save us all some money and include a super-easy recipe for this über-popular dish. And my favorite aspect of the dish is that you can top it with almost anything. For this particular recipe, Heirloom has included their in-house granola, so I recommend you make a big batch and save it in your pantry!

FOR THE GRANOLA

4 cups old-fashioned oats
  (not quick-cooking!)

1 cup sliced almonds

½ cup shredded unsweetened
  coconut

½ cup pure maple syrup

½ cup coconut oil, melted

½ cup packed brown sugar

⅓ cup pumpkin seeds

⅓ cup sunflower seeds

2 teaspoons lemon zest
  (from about 2 lemons)

1 teaspoon baking powder

½ teaspoon sea salt

FOR THE AÇAI SMOOTHIE

1 dragon fruit, peeled and
  cut into chunks

½ (100 gram) packet frozen
  açai puree

1 banana, peeled

½ cup almond milk

Fresh berries or sliced fruit of
  your choosing, for serving

1 tablespoon hemp seeds,
  for serving

1   Make the granola: Preheat the oven to 325°F. Line a rimmed baking sheet with parchment paper.

2   In a large bowl, combine the oats, almonds, coconut, maple syrup, melted coconut oil, brown sugar, pumpkin seeds, sunflower seeds, lemon zest, baking powder, and salt. Toss to combine. Spread the mixture over the prepared pan in an even layer.

3   Bake the granola, stirring every 10 to 15 minutes, until golden brown, about 45 minutes. Let cool completely. (The granola can be stored in an airtight container at room temperature for up to 1 week.)

4   Make the açai smoothie: In a blender, combine the dragon fruit, açai pulp, banana, and almond milk; blend until smooth.

5   Pour the smoothie into a deep bowl. Top with some of the granola and some fresh berries. Sprinkle with the hemp seeds and enjoy.

TIP

Top your açai bowl with fresh fruit, nuts and seeds, or your favorite ready-made granola to save you some time in your busy day!

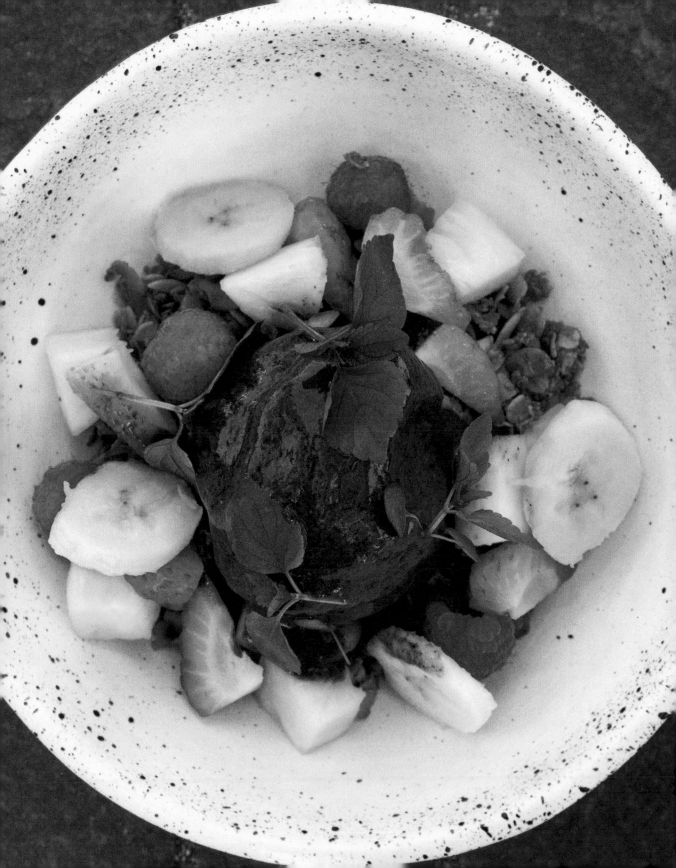

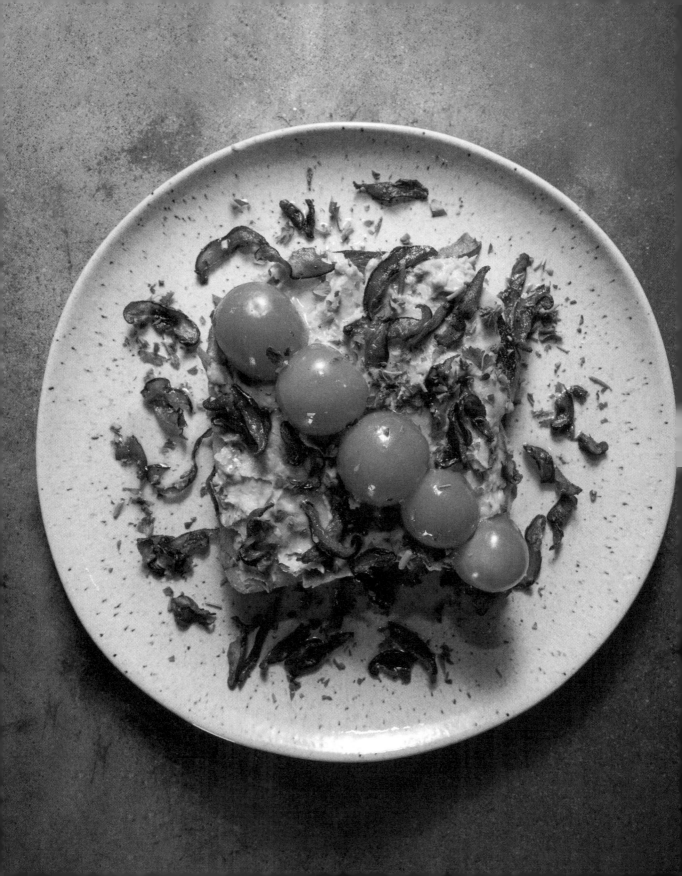

Inspired by Veggie Galaxy in Cambridge, Massachusetts

AVOCADO TOAST

SERVES 2   PREP TIME 10 MIN   COOKING TIME 2 HR (FOR THE BACON BITS)
TOTAL TIME 2 HR 10 MIN, PLUS 1 HR COOLING

Ahh yes, the infamous avocado toast. I swear, when I was in high school, we didn't even have avocados, but as soon as I went to college, they were like that classic pair of Converse Chuck Taylors—everyone had a pair! It was as if I went to sleep one night not knowing avocados existed, and the next day everyone was walking around with an avocado in their hand. I personally love avocado toast because it's loaded with good fats and omega-3s, and one single avocado contains about 10 grams of fiber, which is half the recommended daily intake. I suggest you have fun with this recipe—it's easy to make and so versatile. Sometimes, I just like a simple avocado toast with hot sauce; other times, I like to be wild and add something like dried fruit to it—whatever it is you want to try, you can't really go wrong! But to start, this avocado toast, inspired by Veggie Galaxy in Cambridge, Massachusetts, is a classic you'll definitely want to try.

FOR THE SHIITAKE "BACON" BITS

1/2 pound shiitake mushrooms, stemmed, caps sliced

1 tablespoon olive oil

3/4 teaspoon smoked paprika

Sea salt and freshly ground black pepper

FOR THE AVOCADO TOAST

4 slices regular or gluten-free whole-grain bread, toasted

2 very ripe avocados, halved and pitted

Sea salt and freshly ground black pepper

Olive oil, for drizzling

10 cherry tomatoes, halved

2 tablespoons chopped fresh cilantro leaves

1   Make the shiitake "bacon" bits: Preheat the oven to 300°F. Line a rimmed baking sheet with parchment paper.

2   Combine the mushrooms, olive oil, and paprika on the prepared baking sheet. Season with salt and pepper and toss well. Spread the mushrooms over the pan in a single layer. Bake, stirring occasionally, until the mushrooms are mostly dehydrated (they should be crisp but still slightly chewy), about 2 hours. Let cool completely. (The "bacon" bits can be stored in an airtight container in the fridge for up to 2 weeks.)

3   Make the avocado toast: Using a fork, mash the avocados in their skins until creamy.

4   Spread the mashed avocado over the slices of toast. Season with salt and pepper and drizzle a bit of olive oil over. Arrange the tomatoes cut-side down over the avocado. Sprinkle with the cilantro and shiitake "bacon" bits and serve immediately.

BREAKFAST WRAP

SERVES 4 TO 6   PREP TIME 15 MIN   COOKING TIME 12 TO 15 MIN   TOTAL TIME 27 TO 30 MIN

I honestly wish I had had this recipe when I was in college. We had incredibly long days, and my first class of the day was always at the ass crack of dawn. We started with voice class or Pilates (sounds like the best way to get a degree, I know), and moved on to dance, acting, theater history—the list goes on and on. I often wished I had something I could make the night before, then throw in my bag the next morning to eat on the go between classes. That's why I love this recipe. If you make big batches of each component (storing them in an airtight container in the fridge for up to a week), you can throw this wrap together in about 10 minutes the night before, then eat it on the go, hot or cold, the next morning and get all the nutrition you need for breakfast. It's loaded with protein, packed with flavor, and so nutritious, you'll have enough energy for the rest of your day!

FOR THE PICO DE GALLO

4 plum tomatoes, diced

1 small yellow onion, chopped

Handful of fresh cilantro, chopped

1 tablespoon freshly squeezed lime juice

Sea salt and freshly ground black pepper

FOR THE SCRAMBLED "EGG"

1 tablespoon olive oil

1 red bell pepper, diced

1 small red onion, diced

1 (14-ounce) block extra-firm tofu, drained and crumbled

1 teaspoon nutritional yeast

1/2 teaspoon garlic powder

1/2 teaspoon ground turmeric

Sea salt and freshly ground black pepper

TO ASSEMBLE

2 of your favorite vegan sausage links

4 (10-inch) whole wheat tortillas

1/2 cup vegan chipotle mayonnaise (or plain, if you prefer)

2 cups cooked brown rice or quinoa

1 (15-ounce) can black beans, drained and rinsed

1/2 avocado, cubed

1/4 cup shredded vegan cheddar cheese

1. Make the pico de gallo: In a medium bowl, combine the tomatoes, onion, cilantro, and lime juice. Season with salt and black pepper and toss to combine. Let stand at room temperature until ready to serve.

2. Make the scrambled "egg": In a large skillet, heat the olive oil over medium-high heat. Add the bell pepper and onion. Cook, stirring, until softened and browned in spots. Add the tofu, nutritional yeast, garlic powder, and turmeric; season to taste with salt and black pepper. Cook, stirring, until the tofu is heated through, 4 to 5 minutes. Remove from the heat.

3. Assemble the wraps: Cook the sausages according to the package directions. Crumble them into large chunks.

4. Lay the tortillas on the counter or a cutting board. Spread 2 tablespoons of the mayonnaise over each tortilla. Divide the sausages, rice, beans, avocado, pico de gallo, scrambled "egg," and cheese among the tortillas, then roll each one up like a burrito.

5. Heat a large nonstick skillet over medium-high heat. Place the filled wraps in the pan, seam-side down, and cook until lightly browned on the bottom, 5 to 7 minutes. Serve immediately.

TIP

If you like it spicy, add fresh jalapeños or your favorite hot sauce!

BAGEL & LOX

SERVES 2 TO 4   PREP TIME 15 MIN, PLUS 1 HR COOLING TIME
COOKING TIME 30 MIN   TOTAL TIME 1 HR 45 MIN

If you've grown up as an omnivore, which most people have, then you know how it feels to crave something salty and meaty. And sometimes, I just crave smoked salmon on a piece of toast with some capers. When I moved to Los Angeles, I never thought I would walk into a vegetarian restaurant and find exactly that on the menu—but with carrots instead of salmon?! This recipe satisfies my craving every time, and the best part about it? It's completely plant-based and made using a vegetable you can get anywhere. Carrots: I've never loved your existence more!

4 large carrots

2 tablespoons liquid smoke

4 tablespoons grapeseed oil

4 teaspoons sea salt

4 tablespoons vegan cream cheese

4 slices rye bread, toasted

1 small red onion, thinly sliced

1 tablespoon capers, drained

A few sprigs fresh dill

1 Preheat the oven to 400°F.

2 Place each carrot on a piece of aluminum foil large enough to wrap it. Brush each with the liquid smoke, then let marinate for 5 minutes. Drizzle each carrot with 1 tablespoon of the oil and sprinkle with 1 teaspoon of the salt. Wrap the foil tightly around each carrot and put them on a baking sheet. Bake for 30 minutes. Let cool completely. (The carrot "lox" can be stored in an airtight container in the refrigerator for up to 3 days.)

3 Unwrap the carrots and halve them crosswise. Using a sharp vegetable peeler or a mandoline, shave the carrots lengthwise.

4 Spread 1 tablespoon of the cream cheese over each piece of toast. Top with the carrot "lox," onion, and capers. Garnish with the dill and serve.

TIP

Liquid smoke is strong, so I advise cooking one carrot beforehand, using 1 tablespoon liquid smoke, to gauge your flavor preference before proceeding with the entire recipe.

MAKE IT YOUR OWN

Add sliced avocado or everything blend for a modern twist.

CHOCOLATY SUNSHINE OATS

SERVES 1   PREP TIME 5 MIN   COOKING TIME 5 MIN   TOTAL TIME 10 MIN

One recipe. Ten minutes. Thousands of vitamins and minerals. (I'm not really sure about that last statement, but it definitely has a lot.) I've made this oatmeal more than I've made my bed. Almost every morning of the five years I've been plant-based has started with this exact oatmeal. All the ingredients are raw and, with the exception of boiling water, there is no cooking required. I am honestly convinced Kanzi the bonobo could make this oatmeal. (If you have no idea who I'm talking about, open up YouTube and search "Kanzi the bonobo" right now!) My point is, anyone can make this oatmeal. It takes 10 minutes and it's absolutely packed with nutrients. No more excuses for not eating a healthy breakfast!

½ cup gluten-free quick-cooking oats

1 ¼ cups boiling water

1 tablespoon natural peanut butter

1 tablespoon pure maple syrup

1 tablespoon goji berries

1 tablespoon cacao nibs

1 tablespoon unsweetened cocoa powder

1 teaspoon poppy seeds

1 teaspoon chia seeds

Handful of blueberries, for topping

1 banana, sliced, for topping

1   Put the oatmeal in your favorite bowl and pour the boiling water over it evenly. Cover with a plate and let stand for 5–7 minutes.

2   Add the peanut butter, maple syrup, goji berries, cacao nibs, cocoa powder, poppy seeds, and chia seeds and stir well until all the ingredients are mixed thoroughly, making sure to really mix in the peanut butter and maple syrup.

3   Top the oatmeal with the blueberries and banana and enjoy.

TIPS

Try cinnamon and raisins instead of cocoa powder, nibs, and goji berries for a completely different flavor!

Blueberries and banana are my personal favorites for topping this oatmeal, but you can use whatever fruit you like.

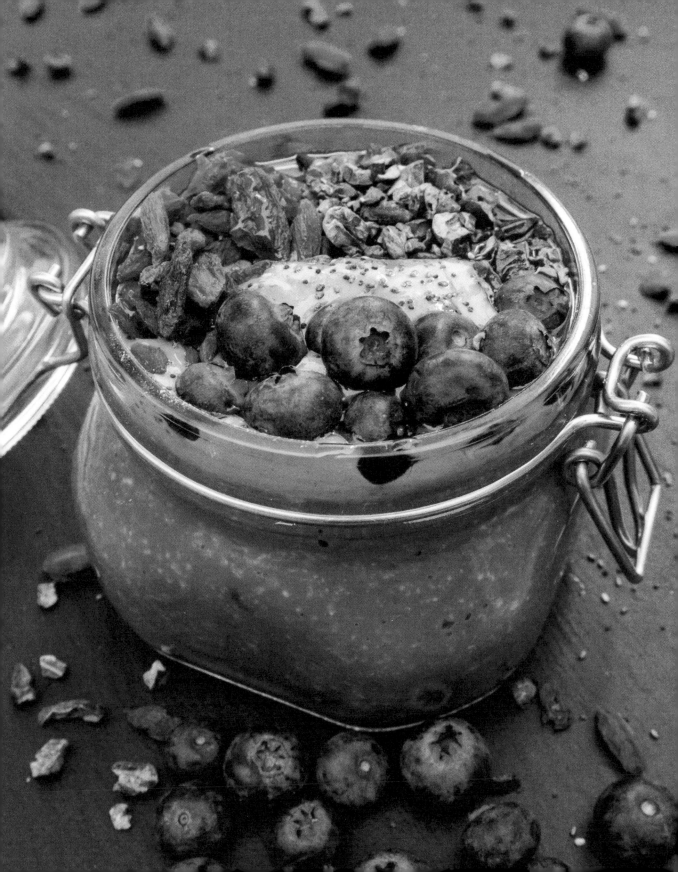

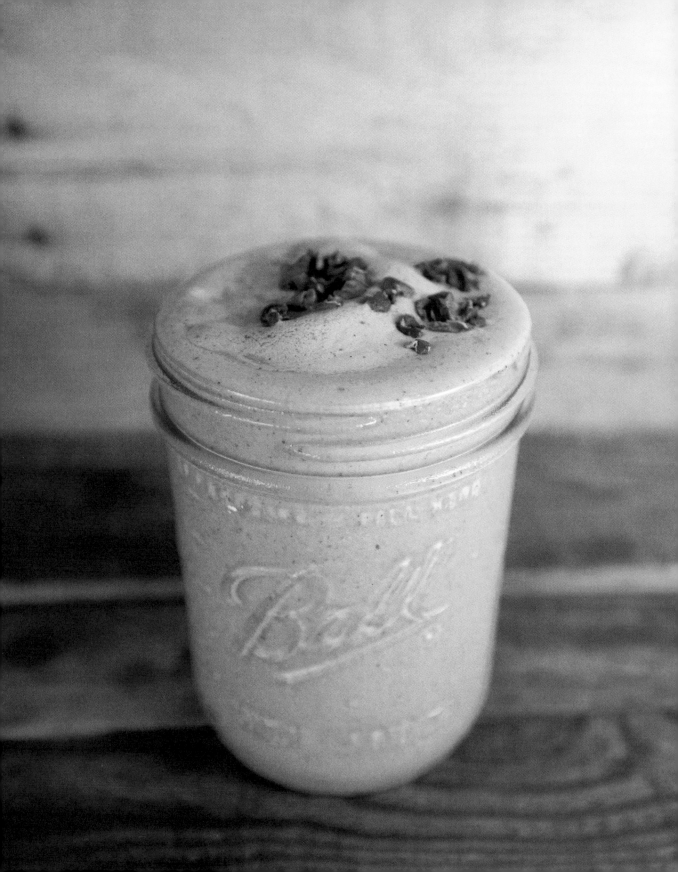

DRAGON FRUIT SMOOTHIE

SERVES 2 PREP TIME 10 MIN TOTAL TIME 11 MIN

I often find myself so busy that I forget to eat or drink anything at all (including water, but that's a whole different discussion). We live in such a fast-paced world that no matter how much we love cooking or how diligent we are about being healthy, we all need recipes that are nutritious and beautiful to look at, which can be made quickly and taken on the go. That is why I am so glad I discovered this recipe when visiting Trilogy Sanctuary in San Diego. This smoothie is packed with vitamin C, potassium, and iron, and you can make it in about 10 minutes—not to mention that it's just gorgeous to look at. I truly believe that when we eat beautiful food, our energy centers open up and expand. What the hell that means exactly, I don't know, but I think you feel better about yourself when you eat beautiful food, okay?! I recommend using an unflavored protein powder for this recipe, but vanilla works well, too, because you're only using two tablespoons to give the smoothie a thicker texture. Combine, blend, and enjoy!

1 large banana, cut into chunks

6 strawberries

1 dragon fruit, peeled and cut into chunks

2 dates, pitted

2 tablespoons protein powder

3 tablespoons natural almond butter

1 ½ cups coconut milk

½ teaspoon cacao nibs (optional)

Combine the banana, strawberries, dragon fruit, dates, protein powder, almond butter, and coconut milk in a blender. Blend on high speed until smooth. Divide the smoothie between two glasses, top with the cacao nibs, if desired, and serve.

TIP

If you like your smoothies to have a thicker consistency, use frozen fruit instead of fresh. Buy fresh dragon fruit, peel it and cut it into chunks, then spread them out on a parchment-lined baking sheet. Freeze the dragon fruit until firm, then transfer it to a zip-top bag or airtight container and store it in the freezer to use as needed. You can do the same with bananas and strawberries; peel bananas and trim the tops from strawberries before freezing them.

FUN FACT

Only need one serving? Pour the remaining smoothie into ice pop molds and freeze for a better-for-you sweet treat or fun breakfast on the go.

BLUEBERRY MUFFINS

MAKES 12   **PREP TIME** 15 MIN   **COOKING TIME** 20 MIN   **TOTAL TIME** 35 MIN

One of the coolest things about the food tour I took across North America was all the insanely interesting people I met along the way. No one was more badass than Doron Petersan—a *Cupcake Wars* champion, ultimate baker, and owner of not only her own bakery but also a hip diner in Washington, DC. Her energy, spunk, and passion are unforgettable and contribute to the incomparable atmosphere of her restaurants. This woman rocks, to say the least! I had the pleasure of getting in the kitchen, throwing on my apron, and baking two of her favorite recipes with her. This was one of those recipes, a perfect on-the-go breakfast or snack, and something we should all know how to make: muffins! (See page 156 for the other recipe I baked with Doron.) Even though this particular recipe uses blueberries, feel free to change it up and experiment with different seeds, nuts, and fruits.

FOR THE OAT TOPPING

- ½ cup rolled oats (not quick-cooking)
- 2 tablespoons cane sugar
- 2 tablespoons brown sugar
- 3 tablespoons vegan butter, melted

FOR THE MUFFINS

- ¾ cup nondairy milk of your choice
- 1 ½ teaspoons freshly squeezed lemon juice
- ⅔ cup cane sugar
- ¼ cup lightly packed brown sugar
- 6 tablespoons grapeseed oil
- 1 teaspoon pure vanilla extract
- 1 ¼ cups all-purpose flour
- 1 cup whole wheat pastry flour
- 1 ½ teaspoons egg replacer
- 1 teaspoon baking powder
- ¼ teaspoon baking soda
- ¼ teaspoon sea salt
- 1 cup fresh or frozen blueberries

1   Preheat the oven to 350°F. Line a standard 12-cup muffin tin with paper liners.

2   Make the oat topping: In a medium bowl, stir together the oats, both sugars, and the melted butter until well combined. Set aside.

3   Make the muffins: In a small bowl, whisk together the milk and lemon juice. Let stand for 5 minutes (it will curdle slightly).

4   In a medium bowl, whisk together both sugars, the oil, and the vanilla.

5   In a large bowl, whisk together the flours, egg replacer, baking powder, baking soda, and salt.

6   Pour the milk mixture and oil mixture into the bowl with the flour mixture. Stir with a fork until just combined. Using a spatula, gently fold in the blueberries.

7   Evenly spoon the batter into the prepared muffin tin. Sprinkle the oat topping on top, dividing it evenly.

8   Bake until golden and a toothpick inserted into the center of each muffin comes out clean, about 20 minutes. May be served immediately, warm, or at room temperature.

MAKE IT YOUR OWN!

Try adding poppy seeds, sunflower seeds, pumpkin seeds, finely chopped dried apricots, or chocolate chips in place of the blueberries to see which you like best, or use a combination of different add-ins.

"CHEESY" KALE & BUTTERNUT SQUASH SCONES

SERVES 6 TO 8   PREP TIME 30 MIN   CHILLING TIME 30 TO 60 MIN
COOK TIME 25 MIN   TOTAL TIME 1 ½ TO 2 HRS

When I first transitioned to being plant-based, vegan versions of pastries, like scones, were some of the hardest foods to find. Pastries usually require butter, eggs, cream, and a pastry chef who really knows what they're doing. So you can only imagine how thrilled I was when I found out that my friend Alexandra, owner of Sweet Hart Kitchen, was introducing scones to her lineup. These are not only 100% vegan but they're also loaded with kale and butternut squash so you can feel good about your morning (or late-night) indulgence. Not to mention, you can switch it up and add whatever vegetable, nut, or seed you're in the mood for. Replace the kale and squash with small broccoli florets or sautéed onions and garlic, and you've practically created a whole new recipe. Bake, indulge, and share with your friends!

FOR THE CASHEW "CHEESE"

- ½ cup raw cashews
- 2 tablespoons fresh squeezed lemon juice
- 1 tablespoon granulated garlic
- 1 tablespoon nutritional yeast
- ¼ cup coconut oil
- 1 teaspoon sea salt (preferably pink Himalayan)

FOR THE FILLING

- 1 tablespoon coconut oil
- 1 cup fresh or frozen chopped kale leaves (thawed and drained, if frozen)
- 1 cup diced peeled butternut squash (about ½-inch cubes)
- 1 teaspoon granulated garlic
- 1 tablespoon nutritional yeast
- ½ teaspoon sea salt (preferably pink Himalayan)

FOR THE DOUGH

- ½ cup cold coconut oil, cut into chunks and chilled, plus more for baking
- 2 cups 1 to 1 gluten-free flour blend (preferably Bob's Red Mill)
- 2 tablespoons nutritional yeast
- 1 tablespoon psyllium husk
- 2 teaspoons baking powder
- 2 teaspoons sea salt (preferably pink Himalayan)
- 1 teaspoon granulated garlic
- 1 teaspoon onion powder
- 1 cup coconut or almond milk (not canned)

MAKE IT YOUR OWN!

Use alternative fillings, like sautéed broccoli, roasted red pepper, or sautéed onion.

1. Make the cashew "cheese": Place all of the ingredients in a blender and blend until smooth. Pour into a small bowl and let set for 15 to 20 minutes.

2. Make the filling: In a medium skillet, melt the coconut oil over medium-high heat. Add the kale, squash, garlic, nutritional yeast, and salt. Cook, stirring occasionally, until the kale is tender and the squash is golden in spots, about 10 minutes. Set aside to cool for 15 minutes.

3. Meanwhile, make the dough: In a small saucepan over medium heat, melt the coconut oil. In a large bowl, whisk together the remaining ingredients. Mix in the melted coconut oil until just combined.

4. Put an 11 by 14-inch piece of plastic wrap on the counter or a cutting board. Scrape the dough onto the plastic wrap and press it out into an 8-inch round. Spread the cheese over the dough, leaving a 3-inch border. Sprinkle the filling over the cheese. Fold the edges of dough over the filling to cover it completely and press the edges to seal. Wrap in the plastic wrap and freeze until firm but not frozen, 30 to 60 minutes.

5. When ready to bake, preheat the oven to 375°F with a rack placed in the upper third of the oven.

6. Cut the filled dough, like cutting a pizza, into 8 wedges. Place on an ungreased baking sheet. Bake on the top rack until golden, 25 to 30 minutes.

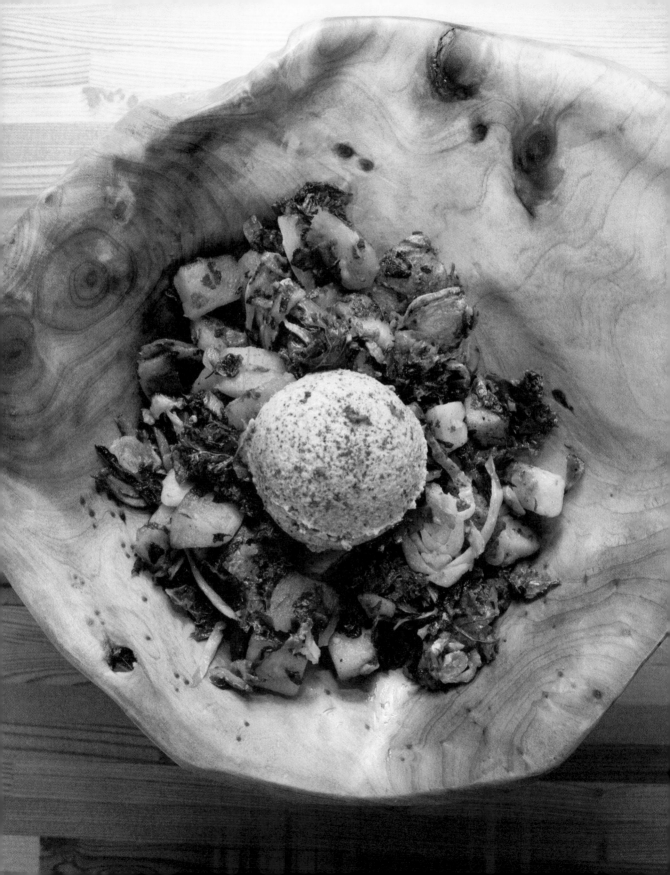

"HASHTASTIC" POTATO HASH WITH CASHEW CHEESE

SERVES 4   PREP TIME 15 MIN, PLUS OVERNIGHT SOAKING
COOKING TIME ABOUT 30 MIN   TOTAL TIME ABOUT 45 MIN

Off The Griddle is a beautiful diner in Portland, Oregon, that started off as a burger cart. Their humble beginnings really influence the kind of food they serve, and all their dishes are super flavorful and easy to replicate at home. I fell in love with this dish because it's exactly the kind of recipe I was missing from my brunch repertoire. It'll give you that carb-y satisfaction you look for on a morning when you wake up a little later after a night out and all you desperately want is something to absorb your hungover-ness. And right on top is a massive dollop of garlicky, peppery cashew ricotta that's the perfect partner to all those potatoes. Pair this dish with vegan "eggs and bacon" or any sandwich you love, and you'll have the perfect brunch! My recommendation is to pair it with another Off The Griddle favorite: the Toasted Jackfruit Tuna Sandwich (page 85).

FOR THE POTATO HASH

2 pounds russet potatoes, cubed

1 pound peeled, cubed butternut squash

1 yellow onion, diced

2 tablespoons olive oil

1 teaspoon sea salt

1/2 teaspoon freshly ground black pepper

1/2 pound Brussels sprouts, shaved

1/4 bunch green curly kale, stemmed, leaves chopped

2 garlic cloves, chopped

FOR THE CASHEW RICOTTA

1 cup raw cashews, soaked in water to cover overnight and drained

1 garlic clove

1 tablespoon freshly squeezed lemon juice

1 tablespoon nutritional yeast

2 teaspoons dried basil

1/2 teaspoon sea salt

Pinch of freshly ground black pepper

A few pinches of smoked paprika, for garnish

1 Make the potato hash: Preheat the oven to 450°F.

2 On a rimmed baking sheet, toss the potatoes, squash, onion, olive oil, salt, and pepper together. Roast until the vegetables are browned on the bottom and slightly tender, 12 to 15 minutes.

3 Add the Brussels sprouts, kale, and garlic to the baking sheet and toss to combine. Roast until the vegetables are browned in spots and the potatoes are tender, about 15 minutes more.

4 Meanwhile, make the cashew ricotta: In a food processor, combine the soaked cashews, 1/3 cup water, the garlic, lemon juice, nutritional yeast, basil, salt, and pepper. Pulse a few times to break down the cashews, then process until the cashews are mostly ground but the mixture still has some texture, similar to the slight graininess of ricotta.

5 Spoon the potato hash into bowls and top each with a scoop of the cashew ricotta. Garnish with a pinch of paprika and serve.

LOADED PANCAKES

MAKES 8 (4-INCH) PANCAKES   PREP TIME 10 MIN, PLUS 5 MIN RESTING TIME
COOKING TIME 4 TO 5 MIN   TOTAL TIME 40 MIN

When I was growing up, there were certain foods I just didn't understand, like pancakes. I would always see them in some form or another in commercials, and kids at school would lose their minds whenever anyone said the word "pancake," but I had never tried them. I asked my parents what pancakes were, but they didn't know, either, so they just told me pancakes were "pita bread with sugary syrup." My parents weren't exactly wrong, but I still didn't understand why kids would act like someone just told them they could fly when someone mentioned pancakes. Until I tried them. Pancakes are an American staple, and after visiting Veggie Galaxy, a picturesque vegetarian diner in Cambridge, Massachusetts, I was inspired to create my own vegan version of every American kid's favorite food.

1 cup nondairy milk of your choice

1 tablespoon apple cider vinegar

1 1/2 cups gluten-free all-purpose flour

1 1/2 tablespoons flaxseed meal

2 tablespoons cane sugar

1 tablespoon baking powder

1 teaspoon baking soda

1/2 teaspoon sea salt

1 1/2 tablespoons vegan butter, melted, or sunflower oil, plus more for greasing the skillet

3/4 cup fresh blueberries, plus more for serving

TO SERVE

1 banana, thinly sliced

1/2 pint strawberries, thinly sliced

Banana Caramel (recipe follows)

Dairy-free whipped cream

Pure maple syrup

1 In a liquid measuring cup, stir together the milk and vinegar. Let stand for 5 minutes (the mixture will curdle slightly).

2 In a medium bowl, whisk together the flour, flaxseed meal, sugar, baking powder, baking soda, and salt to combine.

3 Pour the milk mixture over the flour mixture; add the melted butter. Using a fork, stir to combine. Fold in the blueberries. Set the batter aside for 5 minutes (it will thicken as it rests).

4 In a nonstick medium skillet, melt 1 to 2 teaspoons butter over medium-high heat. Add 1/4 cup of the batter for each pancake, leaving space for the pancakes to expand as they cook. Cook until the edges appear dry and air bubbles form on top, about 2 minutes, then flip and cook for about 2 minutes more, until the batter is cooked through.

5 Top the pancakes with the banana slices, strawberries, blueberries, a dollop of banana caramel, and some whipped cream. Serve with maple syrup.

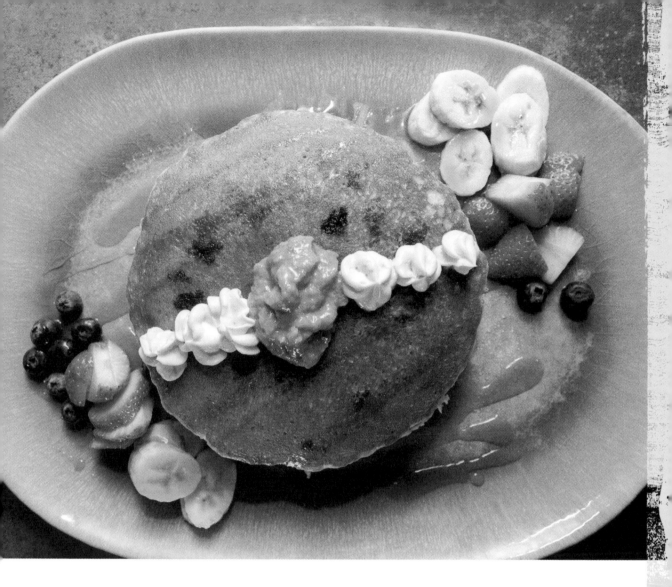

BANANA CARAMEL

1 tablespoon cane sugar
1 tablespoon brown rice syrup
1 banana, coarsely chopped
Pinch of sea salt

TIP
Banana caramel is delicious on toast or stirred into oatmeal, too.

1. In a small skillet, combine the sugar and brown rice syrup. Cook over medium-low heat, stirring, until the sugar has completely dissolved, 1 to 2 minutes.

2. Add the banana and salt, stirring to coat the banana with the sugar mixture, then mash with a fork. Cook, stirring, until thickened, 2 to 3 minutes. Use immediately, or let cool and store in an airtight container in the refrigerator for up to 3 days.

MUSHROOM SPINACH CREPE

SERVES 2   **PREP TIME** 15 MIN   **COOKING TIME** 11 TO 12 MIN   **TOTAL TIME** 30 MIN

New York City has always been known as a mecca for plant-based eateries. When I visited Manhattan back in 2013, it was riddled with the trendiest, coolest vegan restaurants in the world. But now many of those establishments feel old and tired. They're from an older era of vegan cuisine, and many of them have done nothing to keep up with the trends and innovations in plant-based eating. Another borough in New York City, however, has emerged as the new champion of vegan eats: Brooklyn. Little Choc Apothecary was one of my favorites: Located right in the heart of the borough, this quaint two-story café serves up both sweet and savory crepes, made fresh to order right in front of you. And if you're feeling creative, you can even build your own. The mushrooms in this recipe make the crepe feel meaty, and the herbs add so much natural flavor to the entire dish. And once you master the making of the crepe, the possibilities are endless. Make yourself a mimosa, turn on some music, and get creative with this one!

4 Buckwheat Crepes (inspired by Little Choc, see page 173)

2 tablespoons olive oil

1 garlic clove, finely chopped

1 pound cremini (baby bella) mushrooms, sliced

½ teaspoon sea salt

¼ teaspoon freshly ground black pepper

Leaves from 1 (2-inch) sprig rosemary, finely chopped

Leaves from 2 sprigs thyme, chopped

½ teaspoon chopped fresh sage

¼ cup vegan pesto (page 115)

4 tablespoons Cashew Crema (page 41)

1 ½ cups packed baby spinach

1 tablespoon freshly squeezed lemon juice

¼ cup walnut halves, toasted

1. Prepare the crepes, then set them aside on a plate, covered loosely with aluminum foil, to keep warm.

2. In a large skillet, heat the olive oil over medium-high heat. Add the garlic and cook until fragrant, about 1 minute. Stir in the mushrooms, salt, and pepper. Cook, stirring occasionally, until the mushrooms begin to collapse and release their liquid, 6 to 7 minutes. Add the rosemary, thyme, and sage. Cook, stirring occasionally, until the liquid evaporates and the mushrooms are browned, about 5 minutes more.

3. Meanwhile, in a small bowl, whisk together the pesto and 2 tablespoons of the cashew crema.

4. Arrange the crepes on a counter or cutting board. Spoon the mushrooms onto one half of each crepe. Top the mushroom filling with the spinach. Spoon 1 tablespoon of the creamy pesto sauce over the filling on each crepe. Fold the uncovered half of the crepe over the filling to form a half-moon, then fold in half again to make a triangle. Put the filled crepes on four plates, then drizzle with the remaining 2 tablespoons cashew crema, any remaining creamy pesto sauce, and the lemon juice. Sprinkle with the walnuts and serve.

SAUSAGE SHAKSHUKA IN A SKILLET

SERVES 4   PREP TIME 30 MIN   COOKING TIME 35 MIN   TOTAL TIME 65 MIN

Shakshuka is an incredibly popular dish in North African and Middle Eastern cuisine. Every country has a different version, but its essence is eggs and a hearty tomato stew. The key to this dish is the tomato sauce that you soak up with your pita bread as you eat. For this version, Chickpea left out the eggs because . . . well, vegan, duh! But I promise you, with a tomato sauce this rich, you won't be missing the eggs at all. Once you try this dish, you'll have better insight into how people in North Africa have breakfast—they do it up right! We eat with flavor all the time, even for the first meal of the day. And if you really want to be mischievous, cook this up for your non-vegan friends and family and don't tell them it's vegan. In my opinion, if you're cooking, you're entitled to have a little fun!

3 tablespoons olive oil

3 garlic cloves, thinly sliced

1 large yellow onion, thinly sliced

1 small carrot, grated

1 small red bell pepper, thinly sliced

1 jalapeño, thinly sliced

1 tablespoon smoked paprika

1 tablespoon ground cumin

5 plum tomatoes, diced

1 (6-ounce) can tomato paste

Sea salt and freshly ground black pepper

4 vegan sausages

1 cup drained canned chickpeas, for serving

1 tablespoon finely chopped fresh flat-leaf parsley, for garnish

1 In a large skillet, heat 2 tablespoons of the olive oil over medium heat. Add the garlic and onion and cook, stirring occasionally, until softened and golden, 2 to 3 minutes.

2 Add the carrot, bell pepper, jalapeño, paprika, and cumin. Cook, stirring ocassionally, until the carrots are softened, about 2 minutes.

3 Add the tomatoes, tomato paste, and 1 cup water. Season with salt and black pepper. Bring to a boil. Reduce the heat to low and simmer until the tomatoes have broken down and the sauce has thickened, about 20 minutes. Transfer to a bowl and cover to keep warm.

4 In the same skillet, heat the remaining 1 tablespoon oil over medium-high heat. Add the sausages and cook until browned all over, 3 to 4 minutes.

5 Spoon the sauce into four shallow bowls. Spoon the chickpeas over the sauce. Top each bowl with a sausage, garnish with the parsley, and serve.

TIP

This dish pairs well with fresh juice or a good cup of coffee. Best served with fluffy pita bread for soaking up all that delicious sauce!

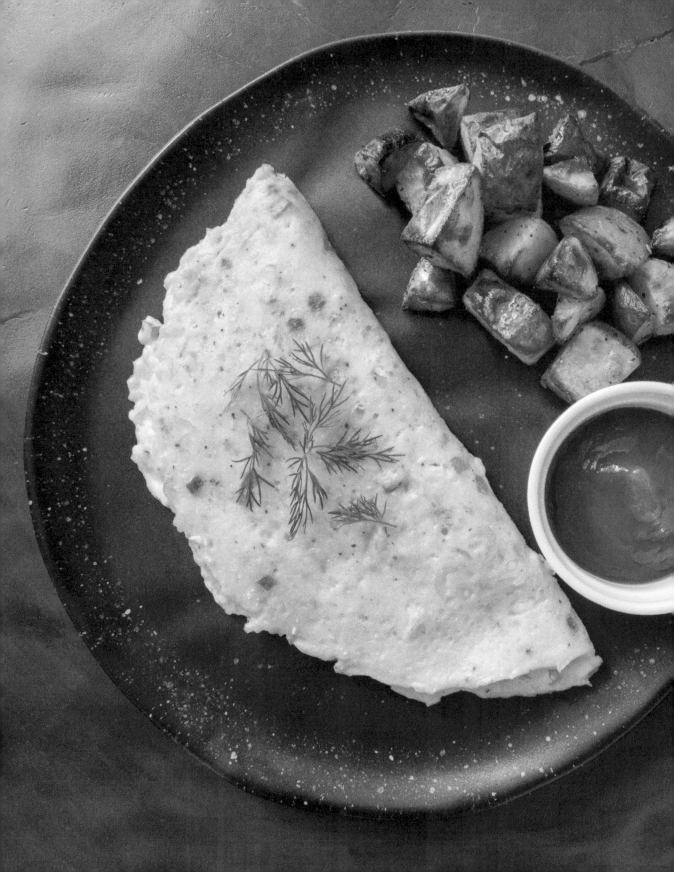

OMELET WITH ROASTED POTATOES

SERVES 2   PREP TIME 10 MIN   COOKING TIME 45 MIN   TOTAL TIME 55 MIN

One of the very first animal products I eliminated from my diet when I was evolving vegan was eggs. I had been doing a lot of research, and one day it just hit me what eggs really were—they're a cavity of hormones that help grow a baby chicken into an adult chicken. And then I started doing the math of all the eggs I had eaten growing up, and that amounted to a lot of hormones! When better vegan egg alternatives started becoming a reality, I was excited to make something I had made often when I was growing up: omelets. And the best part is, you don't have to crack any eggs or whisk those whites and yolks together. All you have to do is put your ingredients in a bowl, mix, and cook!

FOR THE ROASTED POTATOES

1 yellow potato

1 red potato

1 tablespoon avocado oil

1 tablespoon red pepper flakes

1 tablespoon paprika

1 teaspoon ground cumin

1 ½ teaspoons sea salt

1 teaspoon freshly ground black pepper

FOR THE OMELET

¾ cup liquid egg alternative (preferably JUST Egg)

2 garlic cloves, finely chopped

1 scallion, halved lengthwise and thinly sliced

¼ red bell pepper, diced

1 tablespoon finely chopped jalapeño or serrano pepper

2 teaspoons finely chopped fresh dill

Sea salt and freshly ground black pepper

1 tablespoon avocado oil

1. Roast the potatoes: Preheat the oven to 400°F.

2. Quarter the potatoes and put them in a medium bowl. Add the oil, red pepper flakes, paprika, cumin, salt, and black pepper and toss well. Spread the potatoes out on a baking sheet in a single layer. Roast for 45 minutes until golden brown, flipping the potatoes halfway through.

3. Make the omelet: In a medium bowl, stir together the liquid egg alternative, garlic, scallion, bell pepper, jalapeño, and dill. Season with salt and black pepper.

4. In a medium nonstick pan, heat the oil over medium heat. When the oil is hot, tilt the pan to ensure it is coated evenly, then add half the omelet mixture. Cook for 3 to 5 minutes. Flip and cook for 3 to 5 minutes more, until the omelet is cooked through and no liquid remains.

5. Fold the omelet in half, tip it onto a plate, and repeat with the remaining omelet mixture. Serve with the potatoes.

TIPS

Serve the omelet as is or put it on an English muffin to make a breakfast sandwich!

For added creaminess, add two slices of your favorite plant-based cheese before folding the omelet in half and leave the omelet in the pan until the cheese has melted, or add some Cashew Crema (page 41) after plating.

SAN DIEGO

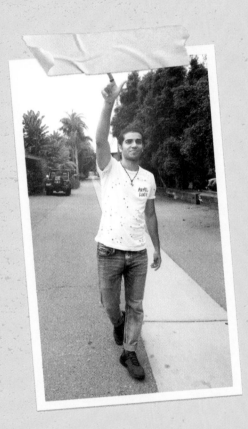

HAVING LIVED IN LOS ANGELES FOR ONLY A SHORT TIME, I REALLY HAD NO IDEA WHAT TO EXPECT FROM THE REST OF CALIFORNIA AND SISTER CITIES LIKE SAN DIEGO.

What I saw on our tour really impressed me. San Diego has all the natural beauty of Los Angeles's palm trees and sunshine but without all the noise and chaos. It overlooks the San Diego Bay, which is a beautiful body of water that runs 12 miles along the coast. After visiting five different vegan spots, I knew that the plant-based scene here was booming! After all, the sheer number of yoga instructors and surfers was enough to justify all the plant-based eateries. But what stuck out to me more than the food was the lifestyle. Without having actually lived there, to me, San Diego feels like living in a small, quiet suburb where all the neighbors know one another by name; instead of malls and buildings and three-story cookie-cutter homes, there's the ocean and palm trees and the sun shining down on beautiful mom-and-pop shops and interesting little bungalows all year long!

It was so clear to me that the vegan community here is really like no other. All the owners of all the plant-based eateries knew one another, and it seemed that all these places were intertwined. A donut shop was recommended to us by the manager of the local vegan grocer, who carried chocolate-covered goji berries from the nearby fast-food chain Plant Power Fast Food, whose founder is also business partners with the restaurateur at a local Southern vegan spot. They all supported and knew one another because they all had one common passionate goal: they wanted, more than anything, more than their own selfish desire to be successful, to help the world evolve vegan.

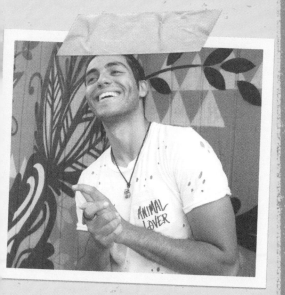

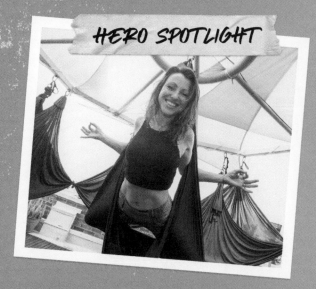

HERO SPOTLIGHT

LEILA DORA
Owner, Trilogy Sanctuary

The moment I set foot in Trilogy Sanctuary, I knew the place was special. There was an energy about it that just took me back to my days in theater school. As soon as I took the elevator up to the rooftop, I was taken aback by the beauty of this sanctuary. And indeed, it was a sanctuary. This yoga studio/superfood café is Trilogy Sanctuary, its name paying tribute to the mind, body, and soul combination that we all strive to master. Owner Leila Dora was a ray of sunshine, and not to mention beautiful inside and out. After Leila met her husband, Roy, at Burning Man (how yoga, vegan cliché, I know), this couple knew that it was love at first sight. And that genuine passion has translated into their gorgeous business. Back in 2014 when Trilogy Sanctuary opened, they took a huge risk by combining a yoga business and a full-service café. But with two yoga studios downstairs, a little yoga shop upstairs, a rooftop patio, and a superfood café successfully serving only plant-based, gluten-free, and soy-free food, Trilogy Sanctuary has proven to be one of a kind—I've never seen anything like it. The colors here, too, are an artistic feat, but the true beauty lies within. Leila roams her spiritual empire with such grace and joy that every diner, yoga-goer, and spiritual guru in the place reflects that same Zen energy that radiates off of her and Roy. And when she decided to teach me a little aerial yoga after our hour-long conversation about plant-based living and the universe while munching on simple and delicious vegan eats, she had my heart. Right there and then, in San Diego, I knew that no matter what it took, there were people out there who were going to strive to make our planet a better place!

CHAPTER 2
APPETIZERS

Featuring recipes from or inspired by:

CHICKPEA
VANCOUVER, CANADA

DONNA JEAN
SAN DIEGO, CALIFORNIA

FARE WELL
WASHINGTON, DC

MAMMA'S KITCHEN

MY HOME KITCHEN

NO BONES BEACH CLUB
SEATTLE, WASHINGTON

PLANTA YORKVILLE
TORONTO, CANADA

ROSALINDA
TORONTO, CANADA

VIRTUOUS PIE
VANCOUVER, CANADA

"CRAB" CAKES

SERVES 4 AS AN APPETIZER OR 2 AS A MAIN COURSE   **PREP TIME** 15 TO 20 MIN
COOKING TIME 30 MIN   **TOTAL TIME** 45 TO 50 MIN

Fish and seafood were the most difficult proteins to cut out of my diet after I eliminated all other animal proteins. They come from the ocean, people don't really know how they are farmed compared to chicken or cattle, and they are easier for the body to digest. Needless to say, their consumption is much easier to justify than anything with legs that roams on land, and because of that, people seem to hang on to them the longest as they transition to plant-based eating. That is why I love this recipe. I rarely crave meat anymore, but sometimes I do want something that tastes like fish and chips or deep-fried calamari or . . . crab cakes! This recipe uses hearts of palm, which are rich in vitamin B6, zinc, and calcium—vitamins and minerals that are harder to find in plants. These not-so-crabby crab cakes from PLANTA in my hometown, Toronto, are a dish you need to add to the rotation!

FOR THE CURRIED DAL

1 cup dried yellow split peas

¼ cup diced red onion
(about ½ small)

1 celery stalk, diced

1 small carrot, diced

2 tablespoons curry powder

½ teaspoon sea salt

FOR THE CRAB CAKES

2 (14-ounce) cans hearts of
palm, drained and rinsed

1 scallion, very thinly sliced

½ jalapeño, finely chopped

1 (1-inch) piece fresh ginger,
peeled and finely grated

2 tablespoons vegan
mayonnaise

1 tablespoon cornstarch

Sea salt and freshly ground
black pepper

2 cups vegan panko bread
crumbs

Neutral oil, for frying

TO FINISH

1 (15-ounce) can full-fat
coconut milk

Small handful of fresh dill,
leaves and tender stems
finely chopped

1 scallion, thinly sliced

1. Make the curried dal: In a medium pot, combine the split peas, onion, celery, carrot, curry powder, salt, and 2 ½ cups water. Bring to a boil over high heat. Reduce the heat to medium-low and simmer until the split peas are just tender, about 15 minutes (for a more traditional dal, cook until the split peas collapse and break apart slightly, about 20 minutes). Remove from the heat, cover to keep warm, and set aside.

2. Meanwhile, make the crab cakes: In a food processor, pulse the hearts of palm a few times, just until broken into large flakes (be careful not to overprocess them); transfer to a large bowl.

3. Add the scallion, jalapeño, ginger, mayonnaise, and cornstarch to the bowl with the hearts of palm. Stir until well combined. Season with salt and pepper.

4. Put the panko in a shallow bowl and season with salt and pepper. Shape the heart of palm mixture into 8 tightly packed balls. Roll each ball in the panko to coat completely, then gently flatten the balls into patties.

5. Lightly coat a large nonstick skillet with oil and heat over medium-high heat. Cook the patties, in batches if necessary to avoid crowding the pan, until golden brown, 2 to 3 minutes per side.

6. Divide the dal among shallow serving bowls. Drizzle the coconut milk over the dal. Top with the "crab" cakes, dill, and scallion. Serve.

TIPS

Remove the seeds from the jalapeño before chopping it if you prefer less heat.

The shaped and coated patties can be stored in an airtight container in the the refrigerator for 1 to 2 days before cooking.

From Virtuous Pie in Vancouver, Canada

GARLIC KNOTS

MAKES 16 GARLIC KNOTS   PREP TIME 20 MIN, PLUS 45 MIN RESTING AND RISING
COOKING TIME 15 MIN   TOTAL TIME 1 HR 20 MIN

I absolutely love entertaining, but it can definitely get overwhelming trying to plan a five-course meal for everyone. So when I'm casually having people over to watch the game or for a chill hangout, I want to be able to offer up some finger food that isn't going to take me hours and hours to prepare. And yes! I have done the ol' chips and salsa with some veggies and hummus, but I think anyone venturing into real adulthood has to step up their game eventually—which is why I love these garlic knots. With four different locations across Canada and the United States, Virtuous Pie is satisfying pizza cravings everywhere and, what's more, these soft, garlicky bundles of joy are sure to impress, as well. Serve them with your favorite dipping sauce on the side, and I guarantee the game isn't the only thing people will be cheering for.

2 tablespoons olive oil, plus more as needed

1 pound prepared vegan pizza dough, thawed overnight, if frozen, or use the homemade pizza dough (page 116)

2 garlic cloves, finely chopped

2 teaspoons nutritional yeast

1 teaspoon red pepper flakes

2 tablespoons vegan butter, melted

¼ cup finely grated vegan parmesan cheese

¼ cup fresh flat-leaf parsley leaves, chopped

Sea salt and freshly ground black pepper

Ranch dressing or marinara sauce, for dipping

1. Line a rimmed baking sheet with a piece of parchment paper. Lightly oil a medium bowl. Put the dough in the bowl and let stand at room temperature to take the chill off, about 15 minutes.

2. Divide the dough into 12 equal pieces. Roll each ball into a 5-inch-long rope. Tie the rope into a knot. Place the knots on the prepared baking sheet and brush them with a bit of olive oil (this is to prevent the plastic wrap from sticking). Cover the pan with plastic wrap. Let the dough rise in a warm spot until doubled in size, about 30 minutes.

3. Meanwhile, preheat the oven to 425°F with a rack placed in the center.

4. In a large, deep bowl, whisk together the olive oil, garlic, nutritional yeast, and red pepper flakes to combine.

5. Bake the knots of dough until golden and cooked through, about 15 minutes. Remove from the oven and immediately transfer the knots to the bowl with the garlic mixture. Add the melted butter, parmesan, and parsley; toss to coat. Season with salt and pepper. Serve hot, with ranch dressing or marinara sauce for dipping.

Inspired by No Bones Beach Club *in Seattle, Washington*

JACKFRUIT FLAUTAS

SERVES 4 AS AN APPETIZER OR 2 AS A MAIN COURSE   PREP TIME **20 TO 25 MIN**
COOKING TIME **6 TO 7 MIN**   TOTAL TIME **ABOUT 30 MIN**

I think every foodie has a special place in their hearts for restaurants that began as food trucks, and No Bones is no different! Back in 2014, this spot was operating out of a food truck in Seattle and now has locations in Seattle, Portland, and Chicago. When I first tried their jackfruit flautas, they reminded me of another menu item back in Toronto at the restaurant where I used to work as a server, so I wanted to use No Bones's creation as an inspiration for my own recipe. Flautas are essentially tacos that are rolled up and fried, and so as long as you aren't afraid of frying and have some toothpicks lying around, this recipe is sure to become a favorite. And like many of the recipes in this book, don't be afraid to have fun and play around with this one. After you master the jackfruit, try it with any other filling you can think of!

FOR THE CABBAGE SLAW AND AVOCADO CREMA

- 1 tablespoon red wine vinegar
- 1 tablespoon neutral oil, such as grapeseed or safflower
- 2 cups shredded green cabbage (6 ounces)
- Pinch of cane sugar
- Sea salt and freshly ground black pepper
- 1 very ripe avocado
- 1 tablespoon freshly squeezed lime juice
- 2 tablespoons canned coconut milk

FOR THE FLAUTAS

- 1 cup packed fresh cilantro
- 2 cups shredded jackfruit (from one 20-ounce can, drained)
- ½ teaspoon taco seasoning
- 1 tablespoon neutral oil, such as grapeseed or safflower, plus more for frying
- 1 teaspoon finely chopped garlic
- ½ bunch scallions, thinly sliced, light and dark green parts kept separate
- 2 tablespoons tomato paste
- 8 corn tortillas
- Cashew Crema (recipe follows)
- 1 plum tomato, chopped
- ½ small carrot, finely grated (about 2 tablespoons)

1. Make the slaw: In a medium bowl, whisk together the vinegar and oil. Add the cabbage and sugar and toss to coat. Season with salt and pepper, then set aside while you prepare the avocado crema.

2. Place the avocado, lime juice, and coconut milk in a food processor. Process until smooth. Season with salt and pepper. Stir in water 1 teaspoon at a time until the avocado crema is thin enough to drizzle. Set aside.

3. Make the flautas: Pick the cilantro leaves from the stems. Finely chop the stems and coarsely chop the leaves, keeping them separate.

4. In a medium bowl, combine the jackfruit and taco seasoning.

5. In a medium skillet, heat the oil over medium-high heat. Add the garlic, light green portions of the scallions, and the cilantro stems; cook until fragrant, about 1 minute. Add the tomato paste and ⅓ cup water and stir to combine. Add the jackfruit and stir to coat. Cook until the jackfruit is warmed through, about 2 minutes.

6. Lay the tortillas on the counter. Spread the jackfruit filling over the tortillas, dividing it evenly, then roll them up into cylinders.

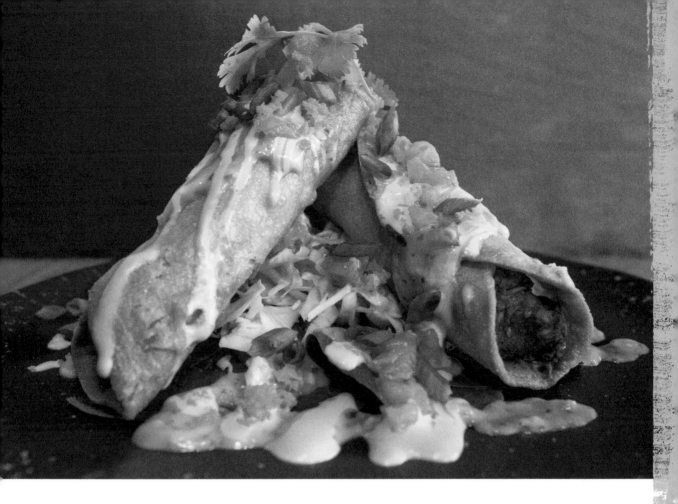

7 Rinse the skillet and dry it well. Fill the skillet with 1/8 inch of oil and heat over medium-high heat. Add the filled tortillas, seam-side down. Cook, turning the flautas occasionally, until golden and crisp all over, 3 to 4 minutes. Transfer to a paper towel–lined plate.

8 Place the flautas on individual serving plates. Drizzle with the avocado crema and some cashew crema. Top with the tomato, scallion greens, cilantro leaves, and carrot. Serve with the slaw alongside.

CASHEW CREMA

MAKES ¾ CUP

1 cup raw cashews

1 cup boiling water

1 tablespoon freshly squeezed lemon juice

Sea salt

1 In a blender, combine the cashews and boiling water; let soak for 20 minutes. Drain the cashews and return them to the blender.

2 Add the lemon juice and ½ cup cold water to the blender. Blend until thick, creamy, and smooth, adding additional water, 1 tablespoon as a time, until you reach the desired consistency. Season with salt.

3 May be prepared up to 3 days in advance and stored in the refrigerator.

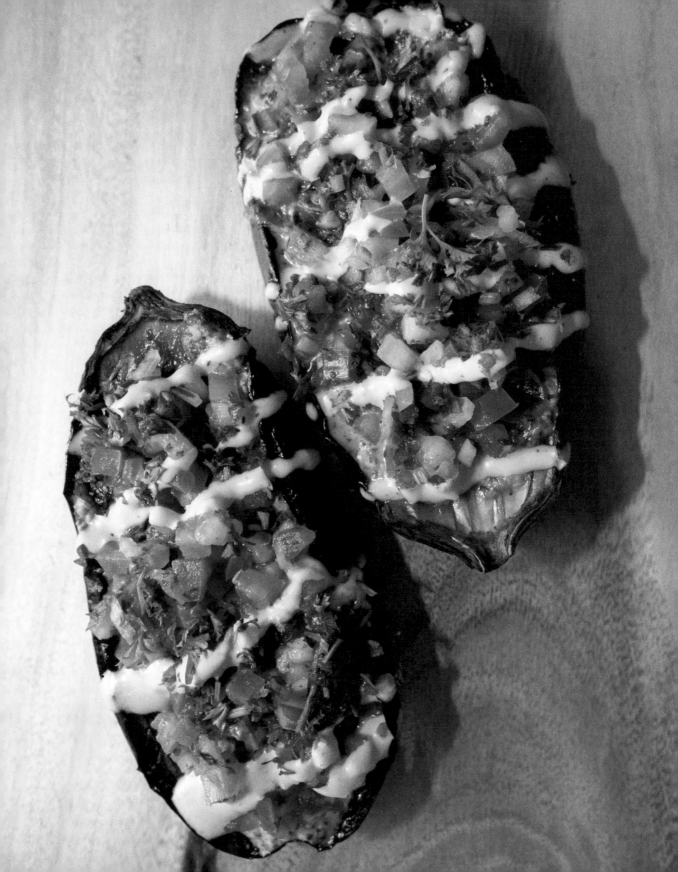

STUFFED EGGPLANT

SERVES 4   PREP TIME 20 MIN   COOKING TIME 25 MIN   TOTAL TIME 45 MIN

If there's one vegetable I never get tired of, it's eggplant. It's super versatile, absorbs flavor beautifully, and is a staple in North African and Mediterranean cuisine. We use it in a few recipes throughout this book, but none are more beautiful than this dish. Mediterranean restaurants are a dime a dozen in many cities throughout the world, but Chickpea really stands out with how it elevates this cuisine. Chef Itamar Shani has a solid understanding of the culinary art that comes out of this region of the world, and he uses that knowledge to create beautiful dishes featuring vegetables—in this case, eggplant—as the stars of the dish. The tomato-mint salsa and green *schug* sauce are components that you're going to want to make in large quantities just to keep on hand in your fridge. So, for more than one reason, I really think you're going to fall in love with this recipe. Instead of saying *bon appétit*, I'll say it in Arabic: *bil hana wish shifa!*

¼ cup olive oil

2 garlic cloves, finely chopped

1 sprig rosemary

2 Italian eggplant (about 8 ounces each), halved lengthwise

Pinch of sea salt

Pinch of freshly ground black pepper

FOR THE TOMATO-MINT SALSA

¼ cup olive oil

2 tablespoons freshly squeezed lemon juice

Sea salt and freshly ground black pepper

2 plum tomatoes, finely chopped

1 small red onion, finely chopped

Leaves from 1 small bunch parsley, finely chopped

Leaves from 1 small bunch mint, finely chopped

FOR THE TAHINI SAUCE

½ cup tahini paste

2 tablespoons freshly squeezed lemon juice

1 garlic clove

½ teaspoon ground sumac

Sea salt and freshly ground black pepper

FOR THE GREEN SCHUG SAUCE

1 small bunch cilantro

1 jalapeño

3 garlic cloves

2 tablespoons freshly squeezed lemon juice

⅓ cup olive oil

1 teaspoon ground cumin

1 teaspoon ground coriander

½ teaspoon sea salt

¼ teaspoon freshly ground black pepper

TIP

Eat this eggplant dish alongside a hearty salad, a bowl of fresh hummus, or simply on its own, depending on how hungry you are!

1 Preheat the oven to 375°F.

2 In a small bowl, combine the olive oil, garlic, and rosemary.

3 Using the tip of a sharp knife, score the flesh of the eggplant halves in a crisscross pattern, being careful not to cut through the skin. Place the eggplant, scored side up, on a rimmed baking sheet, brush all over with the seasoned olive oil, and season with the salt and pepper. Bake for 20 to 25 minutes, until golden and charred.

4 Meanwhile, make the salsa: In a medium bowl, whisk together the olive oil and lemon juice; season with salt and pepper. Add the tomatoes, onion, parsley, and mint and stir to combine. Set aside.

5 Make the tahini sauce: In a blender, combine the tahini, lemon juice, garlic, and sumac; blend until smooth, then season with salt and pepper and set aside. Rinse the blender bowl.

6 Make the green schug sauce: In the blender, combine the cilantro, jalapeño, garlic, lemon juice, olive oil, cumin, and coriander; blend until smooth, adding water 1 tablespoon at a time as needed to thin out the sauce. Season with the salt and pepper.

7 Place the eggplant halves, skin side down, on individual serving dishes. Top with the salsa, then drizzle the tahini sauce and green schug sauce over the top and serve.

MAHSHI (STUFFED CABBAGE, GRAPE LEAVES, MINI EGGPLANT & BELL PEPPERS)

SERVES **4 TO 6**   PREP TIME **45 TO 60 MIN**   COOKING TIME **50 MIN**
TOTAL TIME **1 HR 35 MIN TO 1 HR 50 MIN**

Many cultures around the world claim to have the best stuffed cabbage rolls. Russians, Ukrainians, Poles, and Persians all fight for that honor. The ancient Greeks are thought to have discovered the cabbage back in their era, but seeing as the ancient Egyptians were an older (and more sophisticated) civilization, I personally think that we cultivated the smelly cabbage. I think there's an easy way to settle this, but it has to do with measuring methane gas, and that can prove complicated. Enough about cabbage farts—back to the dish! The Egyptians took the common cabbage roll and decided to stuff many other vegetables, like grape leaves (my favorite), miniature eggplant, and bell peppers, with the same rice mix. The amazing thing about this recipe is that you can use the filling in almost any vegetable that can be stuffed or rolled. If you like spice, I recommend stuffing some jalapeños! For now, though, here are the classic *mahshi* recipes.

FOR THE VEGETABLES

30 jarred cabbage leaves (see Tip)

30 jarred grape leaves, rinsed

2 green bell peppers

4 baby eggplants

FOR THE STUFFING

¼ cup grapeseed oil

2 yellow onions, diced

1 jalapeño, diced

1 (14-ounce) can diced tomatoes with their juices

4 tablespoons tomato paste

Leaves from 1 bunch parsley, finely chopped (about 1 cup)

1 small bunch cilantro, finely chopped (about 1 cup)

½ cup chopped fresh dill

1 teaspoon freshly ground black pepper

1 teaspoon paprika

1 teaspoon ground cumin

½ teaspoon chili powder

2 teaspoons sea salt

3 cups parboiled long-grain white rice

1   Prepare your vegetables: Remove individual cabbage leaves from the jar and lay them flat on a cutting board. Spread the grape leaves out on the cutting board. Cut the tops from the bell peppers and remove the seeds and membranes. Cut the stems from the eggplant and use a spoon to scrape out the seeds, creating a hollow cavity in each (you'll need to remove enough of the eggplant flesh to make room for the stuffing). Set aside.

2   Make the stuffing: In a large skillet, heat the oil over medium heat. Add the onions and cook until softened, 3 to 4 minutes. Stir in the jalapeño, tomatoes with their juices, and 2 tablespoons of the tomato paste; cook until thickened, about 2 minutes.

3   Remove from the heat and stir in the parsley, cilantro, dill, black pepper, paprika, cumin, chili powder, and salt. Add the rice and stir to combine.

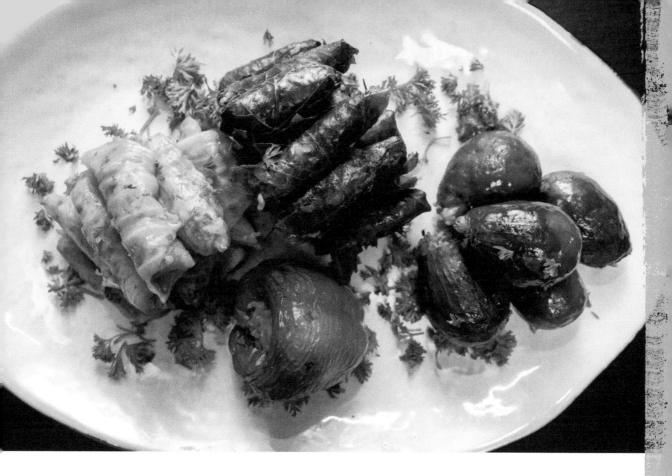

4   In a large pot, combine 3 cups water and the remaining 2 tablespoons tomato paste. Bring to a boil, then remove from the heat.

5   Use a spoon to fill the bell peppers and eggplant with three-quarters of the filling. Spoon the remaining filling onto the cabbage and grape leaves, dividing it evenly, then roll the leaves into cylinders like burritos to close.

6   In a large, deep skillet or pot, arrange the stuffed cabbage, grape leaves, eggplant, and bell peppers, placing the peppers upright (it's okay to tuck them in close). Pour enough of the tomato water into the pot to cover the vegetables. Bring to a boil over high heat, then reduce the heat to medium-low, cover, and cook until the rice is tender, about 45 minutes, adding more of the tomato water as needed if the liquid evaporates before the rice is cooked through. You'll need to taste-test a cabbage roll to determine if the rice is done.

If you can't find jarred cabbage leaves (usually in the ethnic food aisle), use 30 napa cabbage leaves. Bring a large pot of salted water to a boil. Set a wire rack over a rimmed baking sheet. Add the cabbage leaves to the boiling water, a few at a time, and cook until just tender and pliable, 1 to 2 minutes (be careful not to overcook them). Use a slotted spoon to transfer the cabbage leaves to the wire rack to drain and let cool before proceeding.

"MEATBALL" SKILLET

SERVES **4**   PREP TIME **35 TO 40 MIN**   COOKING TIME **40 MIN**
TOTAL TIME **1 HR 15 MIN, PLUS 6 HRS SOAKING TIME**

These hot Italian "meatballs" served in a smoky tomato sauce with creamy vegan ricotta and sourdough bread are another classic from Virtuous Pie. The secrets of this recipe are the sauce and the lemon almond ricotta, so if you're really wanting to make this recipe but don't quite have the time to make the meatballs from scratch, try substituting a ready-made plant-based meatballs. There are many options at local grocers now, and many of them will work just as well as homemade here. I love serving this dish to friends who are coming over for a catch-up and casual hang. This pairs beautifully with an ice-cold beer or a glass of wine, so feel free to make it as an appetizer to serve before a meal or as a stand-alone dish with some *draaanks*! Either way, this recipe should be consumed with friends, and consumed often!

FOR THE RICOTTA

1 cup blanched almonds

Zest of 1 lemon

1 tablespoon freshly squeezed lemon juice

2 tablespoons neutral oil, such as grapeseed or safflower

Sea salt and freshly ground black pepper

FOR THE "MEATBALLS"

8 ounces extra-firm tofu, drained

2 ounces white button or cremini (baby bella) mushrooms

½ small yellow onion

1 garlic clove

1 (15-ounce) can lentils, drained and rinsed

1 tablespoon nutritional yeast

1 tablespoon chopped fresh flat-leaf parsley

1 tablespoon cornstarch

½ cup vegan panko bread crumbs (regular or gluten-free)

1 teaspoon Italian seasoning

½ teaspoon smoked paprika

½ teaspoon red pepper flakes (optional)

Sea salt and freshly ground black pepper

FOR THE SAUCE

1 tablespoon olive oil, plus more for greasing and brushing

1 medium yellow onion, finely chopped

1 red bell pepper, finely chopped

1 garlic clove, chopped

1 (28-ounce) can tomato passata or crushed tomatoes

¼ teaspoon smoked paprika

¼ teaspoon ground cumin

Sea salt and freshly ground black pepper

TO SERVE

Grated vegan parmesan cheese

Handful of small fresh basil leaves

1. Make the ricotta: Put the almonds in a medium bowl and add enough water to cover by 1 inch. Let soak for 6 hours or up to overnight, then drain.

2. Transfer the soaked almonds to a food processor and add the lemon zest, lemon juice, oil, and ⅓ cup water. Pulse until the mixture is smooth and creamy but not pureed (you want it to have some texture, similar to the slight graininess of ricotta cheese). Season with salt and black pepper and set aside. (The ricotta can be stored in an airtight container in the refrigerator for up to 2 days.)

3. Make the meatballs: Squeeze any excess water from the tofu, then crumble it and set aside.

4. Rinse and dry the food processor bowl and blade. Place the mushrooms, onion, and garlic in the food processor and pulse until finely chopped. Add the tofu, lentils, nutritional yeast, parsley, cornstarch, panko, Italian seasoning, paprika, and red pepper flakes. Pulse until the mixture forms a chunky paste (it should hold its shape when you pluck off a piece and squeeze it into a ball). Season with salt and black pepper. Transfer the mixture to a bowl, cover, and refrigerate while you prepare the sauce.

5. Preheat the oven to 450°F with a rack placed in the upper third.

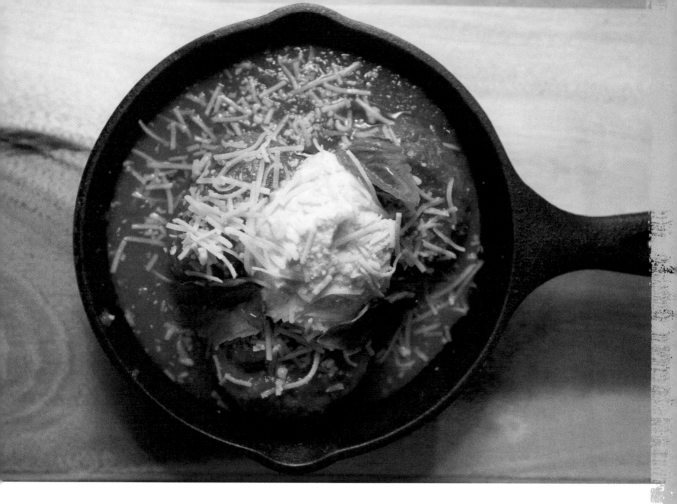

6   In a medium pot, heat the olive oil over medium-high heat. Add the onion, bell pepper, and garlic. Cook, stirring, until softened, 2 to 3 minutes. Add the tomato passata, paprika, cumin, and ¼ cup water; season with salt and black pepper. Bring to a boil, then reduce the heat to low and simmer the sauce until slightly thickened, about 15 minutes.

7   Meanwhile, generously coat a rimmed baking sheet with olive oil. Shape the chilled lentil-tofu mixture into 20 balls. Put them on the prepared baking sheet and brush with some more oil. Bake on the top rack until golden brown all over, about 15 minutes.

8   Add the cooked meatballs to the sauce. Simmer over low heat for 10 minutes.

9   To serve, divide the meatballs among shallow serving bowls. Top with the sauce, a dollop of the ricotta, some parmesan, and basil. Serve.

TIP

Canned tomato passata is essentially strained raw tomato puree. Crushed tomatoes work fine here, too.

POTATO PIEROGIES

MAKES 18 PIEROGIES   PREP TIME 25 MIN   COOKING TIME 15 TO 20 MIN
TOTAL TIME 40 TO 45 MIN

We all love a meal that includes stuffed dough! Whether it be ravioli, a fritter of some kind, or a simple burrito, there is something about sauce and filling wrapped in something carb-y that gets us going crazy! That's why, when I first tried the pierogies at Fare Well (which is owned by Doron Petersan, who also owns DC's Sticky Fingers Sweets & Eats), I knew it had to be included in my book. The best part about this recipe is that once you become efficient at making the dough, not only does the dish become much easier to make, but you can play around with the fillings until the end of time! You can stuff pierogies with pretty much anything and be a superstar chef to all your friends. In this rendition, you will be making a classic potato pierogi, but like I said, feel free to go wild: Sauerkraut and mushrooms, minced "meat" and carrots with parsley, even blueberries are all traditional Polish fillings you can try with this rogue-y pierogi recipe. (I gotta trademark that!)

FOR THE DOUGH

2 cups all-purpose flour

1 ½ teaspoons sea salt

½ cup boiling water

1 ½ teaspoons neutral oil, such as grapeseed or safflower

FOR THE FILLING

4 Yukon Gold potatoes, peeled and cubed

1 teaspoon sea salt, plus more to taste

2 tablespoons olive oil

1 medium yellow onion, thinly sliced

2 tablespoons vegan butter

1 ½ teaspoons chopped fresh dill

2 garlic cloves, chopped

Freshly ground black pepper

TO SERVE

Flour, for dusting

2 tablespoons vegan butter

Vegan sour cream, for serving

1 ½ teaspoons chopped fresh dill, for garnish

1   Make the dough: In a medium bowl, whisk together the flour and salt. Add the boiling water and oil, and stir until a shaggy dough forms; cover and set aside for 10 minutes.

2   Turn the dough out onto the countertop, and knead the dough until smooth, about 5 minutes. Wrap the dough tightly in plastic wrap and set aside to rest while you prepare the filling.

3   Make the filling: Place the potatoes in a medium pot and add the salt and enough water to cover the potatoes by 1 inch. Bring to a boil over high heat, then continue cooking until the potatoes are tender when pierced with a fork, about 10 minutes. Drain the potatoes and return them to the pot.

4   Meanwhile, in a medium skillet, heat the olive oil over medium heat. Add the onion and cook, stirring occasionally, until softened and browned, about 5 minutes. Remove from the heat and add 1 tablespoon water to the skillet; stir to scrape up any browned bits from the bottom of the pan.

5   Add the butter, dill, garlic, and onion to the pot with the potatoes (set the skillet aside—no need to rinse it). Using a fork or potato masher, mash until smooth and well combined. Season the filling with salt and pepper.

6   Bring a large pot of salted water to a boil. If the water comes to a boil before the pierogies are ready to be cooked, cover the pot and reduce the heat to medium-low.

7   Assemble the pierogies: Lightly flour a rimmed baking sheet. On lightly floured counter or cutting board, roll out the dough to ¼-inch thickness. Use a 3-inch round cookie cutter to press out 18 rounds of dough (try to cut the rounds as close as possible, since it's best not to reroll the dough scraps).

8   Spoon the potato mixture onto one half of each piece of dough. Fold the unfilled dough over the filling to form half-moons and pinch the edges to seal. Transfer the filled pierogies to the prepared baking sheet as you assemble them.

9   Bring the water back to a boil, if necessary. Add the pierogies and cook, stirring once or twice to prevent sticking, until they float to the surface, about 4 minutes. Drain the pierogies.

10 In the skillet you used to cook the onion, melt the butter over medium-high heat. Add the pierogies and cook until browned on the bottom, 2 to 3 minutes.

11 Serve the pierogies with a dollop of sour cream and the remaining dill sprinkled on top.

PINEAPPLE & SOY CURL WRAPS

SERVES **4** PREP TIME **10 MIN** COOKING TIME **8 TO 11 MIN**
TOTAL TIME **ABOUT 1 HR (INCLUDES 30 TO 35 MIN SOAKING AND MARINATING TIME)**

When I was growing up, my mom made the best-tasting beef tips and served them with warm pita bread. They were so incredibly juicy, and I would use the pita to soak up all that heavenly grease from my plate. Fast-forward five years, and I still have that dish on my mind, so when we went to No Bones, you can imagine how emotional I got when I saw and tasted this vegan take! I wanted to come up with a recipe that reminded me of those days at my mom's dining table, but with a little bit of a healthier twist. My take on the dish I grew up loving will have you licking your fingers after every damn bite. And no! Not everything with pineapple tastes like a Hawaiian pizza.

1 (8-ounce) package plant-based protein strips

3 cups boiling water

¼ cup tamari

1 teaspoon sesame oil

1 teaspoon red wine vinegar

3 ounces scallions, thinly sliced, light green and dark green parts kept separate

1 teaspoon finely grated fresh ginger

¼ teaspoon finely grated garlic

½ cup drained fresh or unsweetened canned pineapple chunks, finely chopped

1 teaspoon cornstarch

1 head Boston lettuce, leaves separated, rinsed, and patted dry

1 Persian cucumber, halved lengthwise and cut on an angle into half-moons

1½ cups shredded purple cabbage

1 avocado, sliced

1 cup Curried Cashews (recipe follows), finely chopped

1. In a medium bowl, combine the protein strips and boiling water; set aside to soften for 10 to 15 minutes, then drain.

2. In the bowl you used to soak the protein strips, whisk together the tamari, sesame oil, vinegar, light green portions of the scallions, the ginger, garlic, pineapple, and 2 tablespoons water. Return the protein strips to the bowl and let marinate for at least 20 minutes or up to 2 hours.

3. Using a slotted spoon, transfer the protein strips to a plate. Whisk the cornstarch into the marinade. Transfer the marinade and protein strips to a medium skillet and bring to a boil over medium-high heat. Cook until the marinade thickens and coats the protein strips, 1 to 2 minutes.

4. Arrange the lettuce leaves on a platter with the cucumber, cabbage, avocado, and cashews. Sprinkle the scallion greens over the protein strips and serve them in a bowl alongside the platter with the vegetables. Assemble the lettuce wraps at the table.

CURRIED CASHEWS

MAKES **1 CUP**

1 cup cashews

1 teaspoon curry powder

1 teaspoon pure maple syrup

2 teaspoons coconut oil, melted

Pinch of sea salt

1. Preheat the oven to 375°F.

2. Combine the cashews, curry powder, maple syrup, melted coconut oil, and salt in a medium bowl; toss to combine. Spread the cashews evenly over a rimmed baking sheet. Bake until golden and fragrant, 6 to 8 minutes. If made ahead, store in an airtight container.

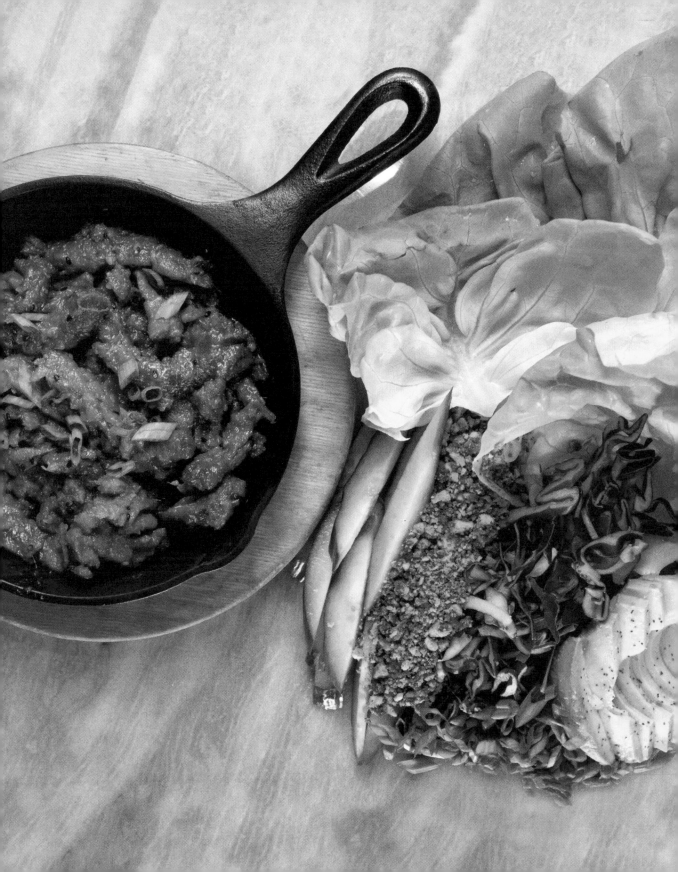

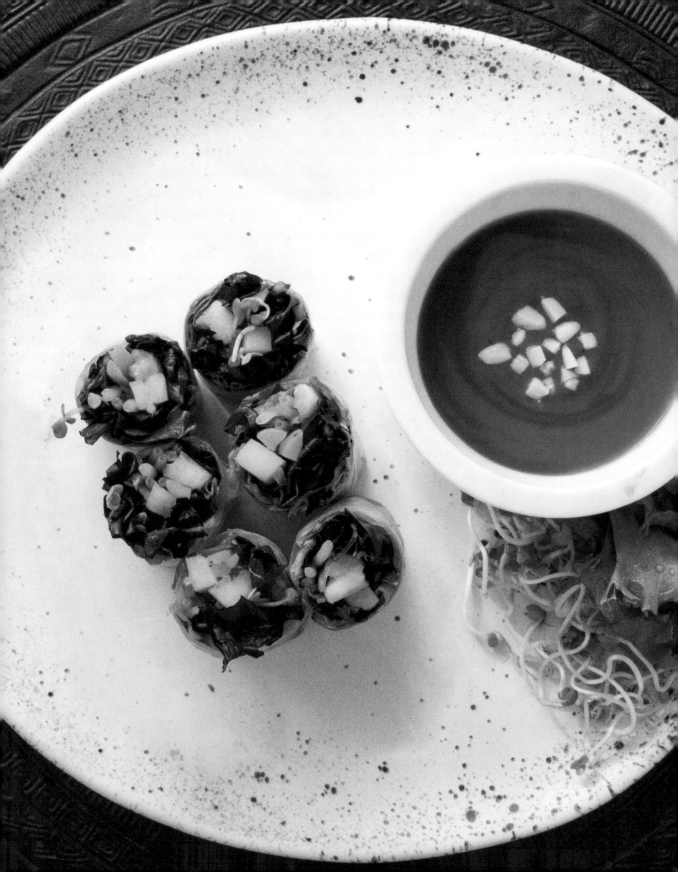

FRESH MANGO ROLLS

MAKES **4**   PREP TIME **20 MIN**   TOTAL TIME **20 MIN**

The first time I ever had a rice roll, it was because of a cute girl. She had ordered them from the menu, and I thought, *Typical. Girl food.* And let's be honest—there's a huge stereotype that exists when it comes to "masculine" and "feminine" foods, but you know what? I CRAVE RICE ROLLS NOW! There's something about these raw, vegetable-forward little packets of vitamins that I love. They're simple, clean, and healthy, and the crunch is so satisfying, it'll have you wishing you were sharing them with a pretty girl (or boy) sitting across the table. And not to mention the peanut sauce. Oh, yes. Nothing like some good peanut sauce on a first date.

FOR THE PEANUT SAUCE

- ½ cup creamy peanut butter
- ½ cup well-shaken canned coconut milk
- 2 tablespoons freshly squeezed lime juice
- 2 tablespoons soy sauce
- ¼ teaspoon finely grated garlic
- Pinch of chili powder

FOR THE MANGO ROLLS

- 2 cups warm (not boiling) water
- 4 spring roll rice paper wrappers
- 4 leaves green-leaf lettuce, sliced into thin ribbons
- 4 radicchio leaves, sliced into thin ribbons
- 1 mango, pitted, peeled, and cut into thin matchsticks
- 1 Persian cucumber, cut into thin matchsticks
- 1 medium carrot, cut into thin matchsticks
- ½ cup broccoli sprouts

1   Make the peanut sauce: In a medium bowl, combine the peanut butter, coconut milk, lime juice, soy sauce, garlic, and chili powder. Whisk until blended and smooth; set aside.

2   Make the mango rolls: Pour the warm water into a shallow bowl. Dip one rice paper wrapper in the water for 10 to 15 seconds, until barely softened (it will continue to soften after being removed from the water, so don't let it soak for long). Place the rice paper on a cutting board. Arrange a quarter of the lettuce, radicchio, mango, cucumber, carrot, and sprouts on the lower third of rice paper. Carefully but tightly, roll up the rice paper around the vegetables like a burrito. Set aside on a plate. Repeat to fill the remaining rice paper wrappers.

3   Cut the mango rolls in half and serve with the peanut sauce on the side for dipping.

TIP

Play around with the vegetables you use for this recipe, or try adding cooked vermicelli rice noodles.

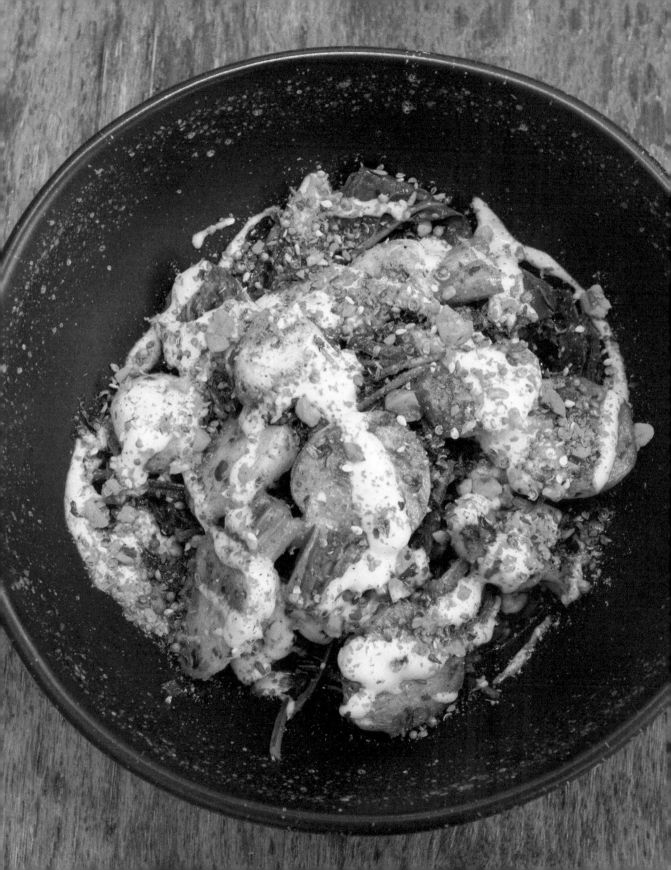

TOKYO TURNIPS

SERVES 2   **PREP TIME 8 TO 10 MIN**   **COOKING TIME 3 TO 4 MIN**   **TOTAL TIME 11 TO 14 MIN**

This dish was the very first one I tried on our tour, and let me tell you, it did not disappoint. Our first stop was San Diego, and on the city's very popular Fifth Avenue strip is a restaurant named Donna Jean, named after chef-owner Roy Elam's mother. Roy wanted to start a restaurant that showed people how beautiful and delicious plant-forward cuisine could be. He focuses on the finest ingredients that come from our beautiful Earth and refuses to cut any corners. He is specific about every single thing in the restaurant, from the beautiful dough used for the pizzas made in-house to the tomatoes they import straight from Italy. His attention to detail has ensured that his customers come back again and again, so much so that they are planning on opening a second location in the vegan mecca of the world: Los Angeles. Whether or not you can get to San Diego or LA to try Donna Jean's delicious offerings is no longer an issue, because now you can make and enjoy one of their beautiful dishes right at home. Tokyo Turnips for everyone!

FOR THE ZHOUG
1 small bunch cilantro

Leaves from 1 small bunch parsley

¼ cup fresh mint leaves

2 garlic cloves

2 jalapeños, seeded, if you prefer a more mild sauce

1 ½ teaspoons ground cumin

1 teaspoon ground coriander

Pinch of ground cloves

2 tablespoons sherry vinegar

1 cup olive oil

1 ¼ teaspoons sea salt

FOR THE TURNIPS
1 bunch baby turnips (with leafy green tops attached)

1 ½ tablespoons olive oil

2 to 3 tablespoons plain vegan yogurt, for serving

2 to 3 tablespoons finely chopped toasted hazelnuts, for serving

1. Make the zhoug: In a food processor, combine the cilantro, parsley, mint, garlic, jalapeños, cumin, coriander, cloves, and vinegar. Pulse a few times to coarsely chop everything, then, with the food processor running, slowly drizzle in the olive oil, stopping to scrape down the sides occasionally. Process until the sauce is smooth. Season with the salt.

2. Make the turnips: Trim the tops from the turnips, then rinse both the turnips and greens and pat them dry. Cut the turnips in half lengthwise.

3. In a medium nonstick skillet, heat the olive oil over medium-high heat. Add the turnips, cut-side down, cover, and cook until browned on the bottom and just tender, 2 to 3 minutes. Transfer the turnips to a medium bowl.

4. Add the turnip greens to the skillet and cook, stirring, until just wilted, about 1 minute. Transfer to the bowl with the turnips. Add 2 tablespoons of the zhoug and toss to coat. (Store the remaining zhoug in an airtight container in the refrigerator for up to 2 weeks.)

5. Spoon the turnips and greens onto plates. Drizzle with the yogurt and sprinkle the hazelnuts over the top before serving.

FUN FACT
Zhoug, zhug, or shoug, as you will see in a few of these recipes, is a green herb hot sauce that is thought to have originated in Yemen. It's gotten so popular that you can now find it jarred or canned at your local grocer. Use any extra zhoug as a spread on sandwiches, as or a condiment for potatoes, or add a dollop on top of your favorite bowl!

YOUNG COCONUT CEVICHE

SERVES 4   PREP TIME 15 TO 20 MIN, PLUS 5 MIN MARINATING
COOKING TIME 1 MINUTE   TOTAL TIME 20 TO 25 MIN

After I graduated from theater school in Toronto, I worked at one of the most popular Mexican restaurants in the city to save up money to move to Los Angeles. I really loved this restaurant and met a lot of good friends there, but the food was just not vegan-friendly. This was a time before the plethora of vegan alternatives and options existed, before what I like to call "the vegan blowup" took place. Many of the dishes at my restaurant seemed easy to veganize, but I guess there just wasn't the demand for it. Fast-forward four years later, and an all-vegan Mexican restaurant is taking Toronto by storm: Rosalinda. This dish is one that I thought would be easy to turn plant-based back when I was working as a waiter because it's essentially a raw dish usually made with seafood. In this case, the scallops, shrimp, or fish usually used in ceviche are being replaced with fresh coconut. The classic Mexican ceviche but made from delicious coconut meat. *Muchas gracias*, Rosalinda!

FOR THE PICKLED SHALLOTS

2 tablespoons apple cider vinegar

½ teaspoon cane sugar

Pinch of sea salt

1 shallot, thinly sliced into rings

FOR THE LECHE DE TIGRE

½ jalapeño, seeded

1 cup fresh flat-leaf parsley leaves

1 cup fresh cilantro leaves

½ cup fresh basil leaves

¼ cup fresh mint leaves

¼ cup olive oil

Sea salt

FOR THE COCONUT CEVICHE

12 ounces fresh coconut meat, thinly sliced (see Tips)

½ small green apple, peeled, cored, and diced

1 Persian cucumber, thinly sliced

1 celery stalk, thinly sliced

Sea salt

½ cup freshly squeezed orange juice

½ cup freshly squeezed lime juice

¼ cup microgreens or pea shoots, for serving

1. Pickle the shallots: In a small bowl, whisk together the vinegar, sugar, and salt. Separate the shallot rings, add them to the bowl, and toss to combine. Set aside.

2. Make the leche de tigre: Bring a medium pot of water to a boil. Once the water is boiling, fill a medium bowl with water and 1 cup ice cubes and set it near the stove. Add the jalapeño to the boiling water and cook for 1 minute. Add the parsley, cilantro, basil, and mint and cook until just wilted, about 5 seconds. Using a slotted spoon, transfer the herbs and jalapeño to the bowl of ice water to stop the cooking. Drain, then transfer to a blender. With the blender on high, slowly pour in the olive oil and blend until smooth. Season with salt and place in the freezer to chill for 5 minutes.

3. Meanwhile, make the coconut ceviche: In a large bowl, combine the coconut meat, apple, cucumber, and celery and season with salt. Add half the orange juice and half the lime juice and toss to combine. Set aside to marinate for 5 minutes.

4. Add the remaining orange juice and lime juice to the blender with the leche de tigre. Pulse once or twice to combine.

5. Pour the leche de tigre into shallow serving bowls. Spoon the coconut ceviche into the bowls and top with the pickled shallots and microgreens. Serve immediately.

TIPS

Check out your local ethnic market for the best coconut meat, usually sold already shelled and peeled.

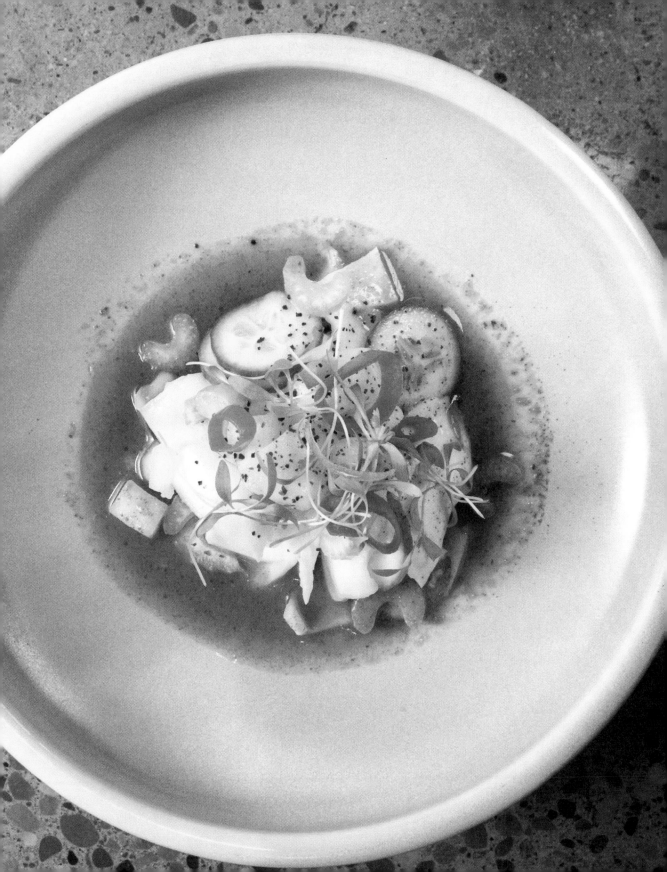

LOS ANGEL

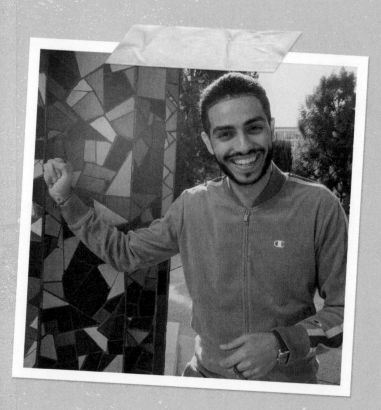

I MOVED TO LOS ANGELES IN 2017.

I had applied for my artist visa and gotten denied, but I applied again and eventually was approved. And I had saved up as much money as I could, because I knew that once I got to LA, I couldn't legally work doing anything other than acting. Needless to say, it was a journey, and it took my blood, sweat, and tears just to get here. Despite all that, when I first arrived I wasn't completely sold on staying. But LA's energy meshed with mine very quickly. I booked Tom Clancy's *Jack Ryan* and worked with John Krasinski, whom I had looked up to for quite some time; tested for my first television series on an American network; and shortly after booked the lead in Disney's live-action remake of *Aladdin*. Los Angeles has been good to me. And not to mention, I was a wide-eyed evolving vegan and had heard of the legends of vegan cuisine in California.

I spent a lot of my free time learning about the plant-based community in

LA and was amazed by the endless choices! Almost every restaurant has a plant-based option or two, but in certain neighborhoods, all-vegan eateries are plentiful: Highland Park, Silver Lake, West Hollywood, and Echo Park are all oozing with vegan restaurants. And while I found out that opening any restaurant in LA is extremely expensive and competitive, these chefs and restaurateurs were more often than not very successful. What makes Los Angeles's plant-based community unique is that everyone in town is a part of it! Even your most carnivorous friend in LA will know about and participate in plant-based eating. Everyone here knows there's no stopping this exploding movement and instead of resisting it, they are usually happy to join in. People here are open to trying new things, and they know that veganism is the future.

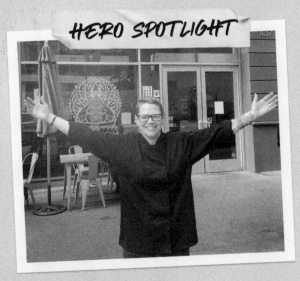

HERO SPOTLIGHT

ALISON CRUDDAS
Owner, Bodhi Bowl

Possibly the nicest person in Los Angeles, Alison Cruddas has been a chef for over twenty-five years and vegan all the while! Originally from South Africa, she moved to the States and had a long career as a private chef. Years later, however, as the vegan scene began to boom, she realized there was a need for a fast-casual restaurant in LA that provided people with a healthy alternative to fast food, especially during breakfast and lunch. And so, Bodhi Bowl was born. I absolutely love this place, and every time I'm downtown, I make sure to grab a burrito or bowl from Alison's super-friendly restaurant. Everything is prepped fresh in-house daily, and with a setup much like Subway or Chipotle, getting your food is super easy and fast.

Alison is one of those rare people you meet who has been committed to a plant-based lifestyle since far before it was hip, cool, or trendy, so she has a lot of interesting thoughts about the whole thing. When I stopped at Bodhi Bowl on our tour, I asked her what her latest thoughts were about the vegan movement. While she thinks the big meat-alternative companies are contributing to the trend, she articulates that what's really impressed her is the number of ordinary people taking a risk and opening plant-based mom-and-pop shops all over the country. For Alison, being vegan is a lifestyle that she adopted over twenty-five years ago, but she says with the recent boom in plant-based products, restaurants, companies, and trends, it's like a new era of being vegan. If you're ever in downtown Los Angeles, make sure to pop your head in at Bodhi Bowl, grab a delicious bowl of plant-based goodness, and say hello! I promise you won't be disappointed.

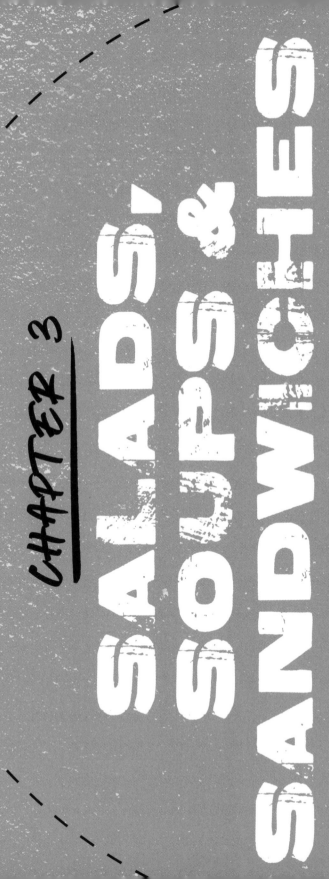

CHAPTER 3

SALADS, SOUPS & SANDWICHES

Featuring recipes from or inspired by:

BODHI BOWL
LOS ANGELES, CALIFORNIA

BROADFORK CAFE
SEATTLE, WASHINGTON

THE BUTCHER'S SON
OAKLAND, CALIFORNIA

FARE WELL
WASHINGTON, DC

INDIGO AGE CAFE
VANCOUVER, CANADA

MEET RESTAURANT
VANCOUVER, CANADA

MAMMA'S KITCHEN

MY HOME KITCHEN

MISSION SQUARE MARKET
SAN DIEGO, CALIFORNIA

OFF THE GRIDDLE
PORTLAND, OREGON

PEACE PIES
SAN DIEGO, CALIFORNIA

PURA VITA
LOS ANGELES, CALIFORNIA

THE SUDRA
PORTLAND, OREGON

WETHETRILLIONS
SAN FRANCISCO, CALIFORNIA

YAMCHOPS
TORONTO, CANADA

KARMA SOBA NOODLE EDAMAME BOWL

SERVES 2   PREP TIME 10 MIN   COOKING TIME 15 TO 17 MIN   TOTAL TIME 25 TO 27 MIN

When I first arrived in Los Angeles I was surprised that the downtown core is not as popular as other boroughs in the city. West Hollywood, Silver Lake, Highland Park are much trendier neighborhoods. In fact, ever since I moved here in 2017, I've noticed that downtown LA is a part of the city that is still very much trying to find its identity. And part of that identity are some really rad food spots that are starting to pop up. Whenever I think of downtown LA, I think of Bodhi Bowl, a super-healthy, satisfying breakfast and bowl shop in the heart of downtown LA. With a multitude of different-flavored tofu and seitan options, you can pretty much have any bowl you've ever dreamed of, vegan-style. Alison Cruddas, who has been a chef for twenty-five years, opened this spot because she wanted to offer people a healthy version of breakfast and lunch during their busy days downtown. And this bowl, packed with protein and whole foods, is one of my favorites. Make this for breakfast or lunch and take it to work. And if you want to cook up something nutritious and easy for dinner, this is a necessity!

Sea salt

3 ounces dry soba noodles

Sunflower or safflower oil, for coating and frying

7 ounces extra-firm tofu, drained and cubed

½ cup sweet chili sauce

4 wonton wrappers, cut into thin strips

FOR THE SESAME-GINGER DRESSING

1 ½ tablespoons sunflower oil

½ teaspoon sesame oil

1 tablespoon rice vinegar or white wine vinegar

¼ teaspoon finely grated fresh ginger

Sea salt

TO SERVE

½ cup cooked shelled edamame (see Tip)

1 Persian cucumber, peeled and diced

1 small carrot, shredded

1 scallion, thinly sliced

1 tablespoon sliced almonds

1   Preheat the oven to 400°F.

2   Bring a large pot of salted water to a boil over high heat. Add the soba noodles and cook according to the package directions. Drain the noodles, return them to the pot, and toss with 1 teaspoon oil to prevent the noodles from sticking.

3   Meanwhile, generously drizzle a rimmed baking sheet with oil. In a medium bowl, toss the tofu and chili sauce until the tofu is well coated. Spread the tofu over the prepared baking sheet in a single layer. Bake until golden and crisp on the bottom, about 15 minutes.

4   Line a plate with a paper towel. In a medium skillet, heat 2 tablespoons oil in over medium-high heat until shimmering. Add the wonton strips and cook, turning once, until bubbled and golden, 1 to 2 minutes (keep a careful eye on them, as they cook quickly!). Transfer the crispy wontons to the prepared plate and sprinkle with salt.

5   Make the sesame-ginger dressing: In a medium bowl, whisk together the sunflower oil, sesame oil, vinegar, and ginger. Season with salt.

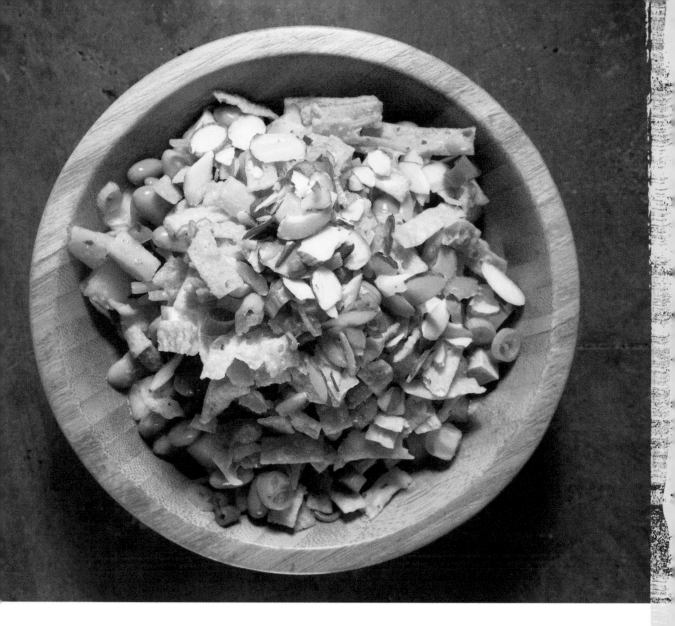

6   Add the edamame, cucumber, and carrot to the bowl with the dressing and toss to coat.

7   Divide the soba noodles between two bowls. Spoon the dessing mixture over. Top with the tofu, crispy wontons, scallions, and almonds and serve.

TIP

If you can't find ready-to-eat cooked shelled edamame, usually sold in the refrigerated section of the grocery store, use frozen shelled edamame and cook it according to the package directions.

SHORBIT ADAS (SPLIT LENTIL SOUP)

SERVES 4 TO 6 **PREP TIME** 15 MIN **COOKING TIME** 1 HR **TOTAL TIME** 1 HR 15 MIN

It gets very cold and gloomy in Toronto during the winter. Temperatures can drop as low as –25°F and states of emergency are often announced because of snow and ice. The best part of growing up in Toronto were the much-anticipated snow days. There's nothing like being a hormonal teenager and waking up in the morning to the radio announcing that school is canceled! And the day always got better when my mom stayed home with us and cooked her split lentil soup. This recipe is super simple, thick, creamy, and delicious, not to mention incredibly rich in protein, vitamins, and minerals. Like any soup, this is best enjoyed on a cold and gloomy day when all you want to do is cuddle on the couch with a warm blanket and watch movies. Or if you simply want something nutritious and light for dinner!

2 cups dried red lentils, thoroughly rinsed and drained

1 large yellow onion, quartered

1 medium carrot, cut into ½-inch pieces

1 medium potato, peeled and cubed

1 medium tomato, diced

4 large garlic cloves, smashed and peeled

2 tablespoons sunflower or safflower oil

2 shallots, thinly sliced

2 tablespoons sea salt

1 tablespoon ground cumin

1 ½ teaspoons freshly ground black pepper

1. In a large pot, combine the lentils, onion, carrot, potato, tomato, garlic, and 5 cups water. Bring to a boil over high heat, then reduce the heat to medium-low and simmer until the lentils have collapsed and the vegetables are very tender (they should be soft enough to easily puree). Keep an eye on the water level, adding more as needed if too much evaporates before the lentils and vegetables are done (the mixture should be slightly brothy but not soupy). Remove from the heat and let cool slightly, about 10 minutes.

2. Meanwhile, line a plate with a paper towel. In a medium nonstick skillet, heat the oil over medium-high heat until shimmering. Add the shallots, in batches, and cook until deep golden and crisp, about 8 minutes. Using a slotted spoon, transfer the shallots to the prepared plate to drain.

3. In batches, carefully transfer the soup to a blender and blend until smooth. Return the soup to the pot, add the salt, cumin, and pepper and warm over medium heat, 3 to 5 minutes.

4. Ladle the soup into individual bowls, top with the fried shallots, and serve.

TIP

As an added touch, if you like, quarter a pita bread, drizzle with olive oil, and sprinkle with oregano, and bake at 380°F for 10 minutes per side, then enjoy it with the soup.

FRESH CHICKPEA SALAD

SERVES 2 TO 4   PREP TIME 15 MIN   TOTAL TIME 15 MIN

When I'm working on set, I usually don't have the time or brain capacity to think about anything else. If I have any free time off set in the day, it's usually spent at the gym. And after a hard workout and a long day, I want something that is incredibly simple, packed with protein, and dense with nutrients. That's why I love this recipe. I can whip it up in about 15 minutes using the veggies I have in the fridge, and feel good about what I'm putting in my body. With all the meat and cheese alternatives that exist today, it can be very tempting to just throw a vegan frozen dinner or pizza in the oven and call it a day. But this salad will take less time and provide more protein, and it's much healthier than anything you can buy from the store. So when people ask me, "Where do you get your protein from?" this is a dish I recommend *a lot*.

2 cups drained canned or cooked chickpeas

1 heirloom tomato, diced

1 medium Persian cucumber, halved and sliced

1/2 large avocado, diced

2 tablespoons pitted kalamata olives, halved

1 tablespoon freshly squeezed lime juice

1 tablespoon finely chopped fresh dill

1 1/2 teaspoons ground cumin

1 teaspoon ground coriander

1 1/2 teaspoons sea salt

Vegan feta cheese, for serving (optional)

1 scallion, sliced, for garnish

1   Place the chickpeas in a large bowl. Add the tomato, cucumber, avocado, olives, lime juice, dill, cumin, coriander, and salt to the same bowl and mix well.

2   Crumble the feta on top, garnish with the scallions, and serve.

TIPS

If you're using sprouted chickpeas, I recommend adding a little bit of apple cider vinegar to the salad to cut that earthy flavor sprouted legumes have.

Feel free to substitute lentils, kidney beans, or black-eyed peas for the chickpeas.

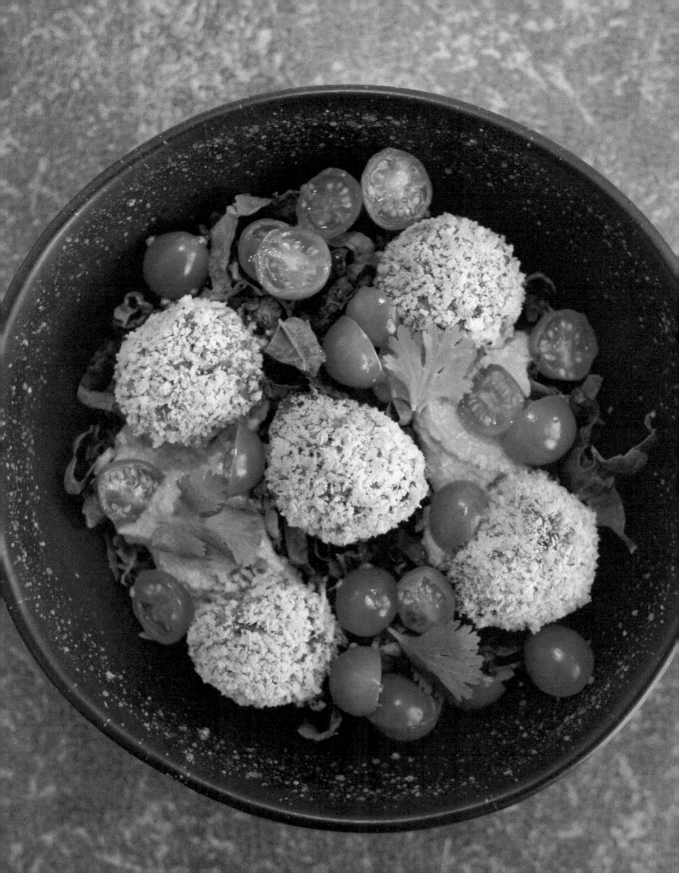

THE CAIRO FALAFEL SALAD

SERVES 2   PREP TIME 20 MIN, PLUS 30 MIN CHILLING TIME
COOKING TIME 43 TO 50 MIN   TOTAL TIME 60 TO 70 MIN

I have tried hundreds of different falafels in my life. Weddings, church gatherings, family dinners, funerals, you name it—if there is a gathering of Egyptians, there is falafel! The reason I wanted to include this one in particular is because I found it to be a little different than any falafel I have ever tried. It's rolled in panko bread crumbs, which is definitely unusual, but to utilize the falafel so it's the star of a salad is something I haven't seen all that much. When I tried this dish as a whole, I really fell in love with it. It takes all the healthy components of the falafel and combines them with other incredibly nutritious ingredients to make a superfood salad.

1 pound Italian eggplant, peeled and cubed

4 tablespoons neutral oil, such as grapeseed or safflower, plus more for drizzling

1/2 cup drained canned chickpeas

1/4 cup cooked quinoa

1 medium yellow onion, diced

2 garlic cloves, finely chopped

1/2 cup packed fresh flat-leaf parsley

Zest from 1/2 lemon

2 teaspoon freshly squeezed lemon juice

1 1/2 teaspoons ground cumin

1 teaspoon ground coriander

3/4 teaspoon sea salt, plus more for seasoning

1/2 teaspoon freshly ground black pepper, plus more for seasoning

1/4 teaspoon cayenne pepper

2 cups vegan panko bread crumbs

1 (10-ounce) bunch Tuscan kale, stemmed, leaves sliced into thin ribbons

1/4 cup jarred romesco sauce

1/2 pint cherry tomatoes, halved

1 Preheat the oven to 400°F.

2 On a rimmed baking sheet, toss the eggplant with 2 tablespoons of the oil. Bake, stirring occasionally, until very tender and browned in spots, 25 to 30 minutes. Set aside to let cool for at least 10 minutes.

3 In a food processor, combine the chickpeas, quinoa, onion, garlic, parsley, lemon zest, lemon juice, cumin, coriander, salt, black pepper, cayenne, and 1 tablespoon of the oil. Pulse, stopping to scrape down the sides as needed, until the chickpeas are completely pureed and the mixture loosely holds its shape when squeezed together; if it doesn't, process the mixture a bit more. Transfer to a bowl, cover, and refrigerate for at least 30 minutes and up to 2 hours.

4 Put the panko in a shallow bowl. Add the remaining 1 tablespoon oil, season with salt and black pepper, and rub the panko crumbs together to work in the oil.

5 Shape the chilled falafel mixture into 12 balls, then roll them in the panko to completely coat.

6 Lightly drizzle the baking sheet you used for the eggplant with oil. Place the falafel on the baking sheet and lightly drizzle with more oil. Bake until golden brown on the bottom, 18 to 20 minutes.

7 Meanwhile, in a medium bowl, toss the kale with half the romesco sauce.

8 Divide the kale between two shallow bowls. Top with the tomatoes, eggplant, falafel, and remaining romesco sauce and serve.

ARTICHOKE & CASHEW CHEESE SANDWICH WITH CUCUMBERS & SPROUTS

SERVES 2   PREP TIME 20 MIN   COOKING TIME 3 TO 5 MIN   TOTAL TIME 23 TO 25 MIN

You know when you were a kid and you came home from school and were just starving? To shut me up, my mom used to make me fries, throw them in some pita bread, and tell me to eat my sandwich and be quiet until dinner. A sandwich made from fries, Mom?! Really? But it truly was a popular practice among Egyptian moms. The reason I love *this* recipe is because I think I'm a little too old (and maybe too sophisticated) to be eating a fry sandwich, but this feels like an elevated version of the snack my mom used to make me before dinner. And if you really want to experience what it was like to be little old me, feel free to switch out the artichokes for cooked sunchokes, because you'll be surprised to how similar they are to potatoes.

FOR THE ARTICHOKE SPREAD

1 (14-ounce) can artichoke hearts packed in water, drained

1 garlic clove

1 tablespoon apple cider vinegar

½ teaspoon sea salt

3 tablespoons olive oil

Leaves from 1 small bunch flat-leaf parsley, chopped

FOR THE CHEESY CASHEW SPREAD

1 cup cashews

1 tablespoon nutritional yeast

¼ teaspoon sea salt

¼ teaspoon garlic powder

¼ teaspoon onion powder

Pinch of ground turmeric

Pinch of ground nutmeg

FOR THE SANDWICHES

2 tablespoons vegan mayonnaise

4 slices sourdough bread

1 Persian cucumber, thinly sliced

1 cup alfalfa or broccoli sprouts

1   Make the artichoke spread: In a food processor, combine the artichoke hearts, garlic, vinegar, and salt. With the food processor running, drizzle in the olive oil and process until the mixture is pureed. Transfer to a medium bowl and stir in the parsley.

2   Make the cheesy cashew spread: Rinse and dry the food processor bowl and blade. Place the cashews, nutritional yeast, salt, garlic powder, onion powder, turmeric, nutmeg, and ¼ cup water in the food processor. Pulse until the mixture is smooth, adding additional water 1 tablespoon at a time, if needed.

3   Make the sandwiches: Heat a large nonstick skillet over medium heat. Spread the mayonnaise over one side of each slice of bread. Spread some of the artichoke spread over the other side of two slices of the bread and some of the cashew spread over the other side of the remaining two slices (save any remaining artichoke spread and cheesy cashew spread for another use).

4   Put the bread, mayo-side down, in the skillet. Cook until deep golden and crisp on the bottom, 3 to 5 minutes.

5   Transfer the artichoke-topped bread to individual plates. Divide the cucumbers and sprouts between them. Top each with a slice of the cashew-cheese-topped bread, mayo-side up, to close the sandwiches. Serve immediately.

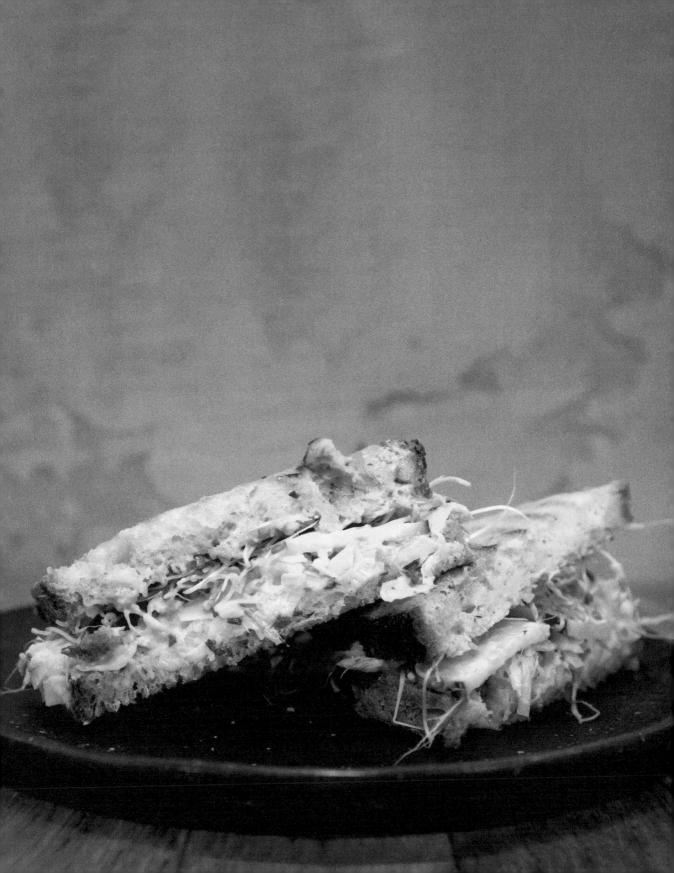

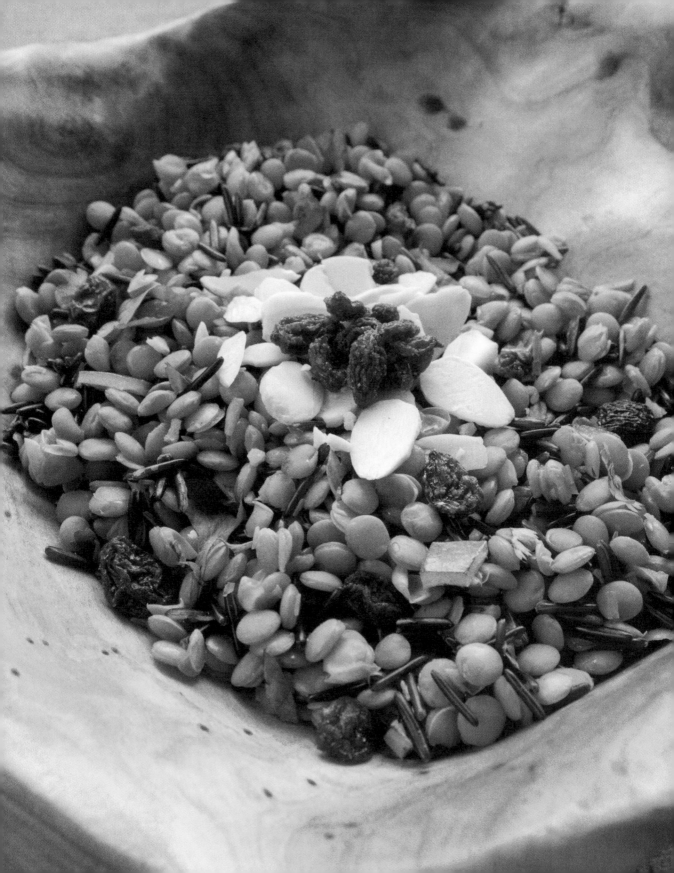

From Mamma's Kitchen

GREEN LENTIL SALAD

SERVES 2 TO 4   PREP TIME 10 MIN, PLUS 15 MIN CHILLING TIME
COOKING TIME 45 MIN   TOTAL TIME 1 HR 10 MIN

My mom doesn't frequently add new recipes to her repertoire, but for some reason, over the past few years, this one has just stuck. It uses the lentil—an ingredient she is incredibly familiar with and one that is very common in North African cuisine—but in a completely different way. This salad is bursting with protein, so I love to make it during weeks when I know I will be training especially hard. I always make a big batch and use it to supplement the majority of my meals, and it satisfies the cravings I often find myself having for that "salty and sweet" combination. The best part about it—apart from the rice and lentils— is that there isn't really any cooking involved. Just a great combination of whole, fresh ingredients that will have you feeling like a superstar!

1 cup dried wild rice, rinsed and drained

1 teaspoon sea salt

½ cup dried French or green lentils, picked over, rinsed, and drained

¼ cup apple cider vinegar

1 teaspoon ground coriander

1 teaspoon ground cumin

½ teaspoon ground turmeric

¼ teaspoon ground cinnamon

1 medium red onion, diced

½ cup sliced almonds, toasted

½ cup chopped fresh flat-leaf parsley leaves

¼ cup dried currants

¼ cup olive oil

¼ teaspoon freshly ground black pepper

1. In a medium pot, combine the wild rice, ¾ teaspoon of the salt, and 4 cups water. Bring to a boil over medium-high heat. Reduce to a simmer and continue cooking until the rice is tender, about 45 minutes. Drain the rice.

2. Meanwhile, in a small pot, combine the lentils and 1 ½ cups water and bring to a boil. Reduce the heat to medium-low and simmer until tender, 20 to 25 minutes. Drain any excess water.

3. Once the rice and lentils are cooked, in a medium bowl, whisk together the vinegar, coriander, cumin, turmeric, and cinnamon. Add the rice, lentils, onion, almonds, parsley, currants, and olive oil. Stir to combine, then season with the remaining ¼ teaspoon salt and the pepper. Refrigerate for at least 15 minutes or up to overnight before serving.

TIPS

Substitute 1 (15-ounce) can cooked lentils (drained and rinsed) as a shortcut.

Raisins can be subbed in for the currants.

GIAMBOTTA STEW

SERVES 4   PREP TIME 20 MIN   COOKING TIME 23 TO 27 MIN   TOTAL TIME 43 TO 47 MIN

I love this dish because it's a high-protein recipe that you can feel good about eating often. And with Pura Vita's Chef Tara behind it, you know it's going to taste like it came straight from your (or your friend's) Italian nonna's kitchen. Filled with fresh vegetables and chickpeas, this may be the most nutritious recipe in the whole book! The key to the dish is the tomatoes. In most recipes, it doesn't really matter what tomatoes you use—though I always think the better-quality ingredients you use, the better the outcome—but for this dish especially, I would recommend a quality whole peeled tomato like Chef Tara suggests. Serve it on its own or as a side with a sandwich, and there's no going wrong with this one.

3 tablespoons olive oil

1 medium yellow onion, diced

2 celery stalks, diced

2 carrots, diced

1 Italian eggplant (about 8 ounces), peeled and diced (see Tip)

1 red bell pepper, diced

2 garlic cloves, chopped

¼ teaspoon red pepper flakes

Sea salt and freshly ground black pepper

1 (20-ounce) can whole peeled tomatoes

4 Yukon Gold potatoes, peeled and cubed

1 medium zucchini, diced

1 cup drained canned chickpeas

1 bay leaf, preferably fresh

1 teaspoon chopped fresh thyme leaves

1 teaspoon chopped fresh tarragon

¼ cup chopped fresh flat-leaf parsley

¼ cup fresh basil leaves, torn into small pieces

Toasted ciabatta bread, for serving

1 In a large pot, heat 2 tablespoons of the olive oil over medium-high heat. Add the onion, celery, carrots, eggplant, bell pepper, garlic, and red pepper flakes; season with salt and black pepper. Cook, stirring occasionally, until the vegetables are golden and softened, 8 to 10 minutes.

2 Meanwhile, finely chop the tomatoes in the can using kitchen shears (alternatively, pulse them in a food processor until chopped but still chunky). Add the tomatoes to the pot with the vegetables and bring to a boil.

3 Add the potatoes, zucchini, chickpeas, bay leaf, thyme, and tarragon. Reduce the heat to medium and simmer until the potatoes are tender but not falling apart, 10 to 12 minutes.

4 Stir in the parsley and basil. Spoon into bowls, drizzle with the remaining 1 tablespoon oil, and serve with toasted ciabatta.

TIP

You can substitute Japanese eggplant.

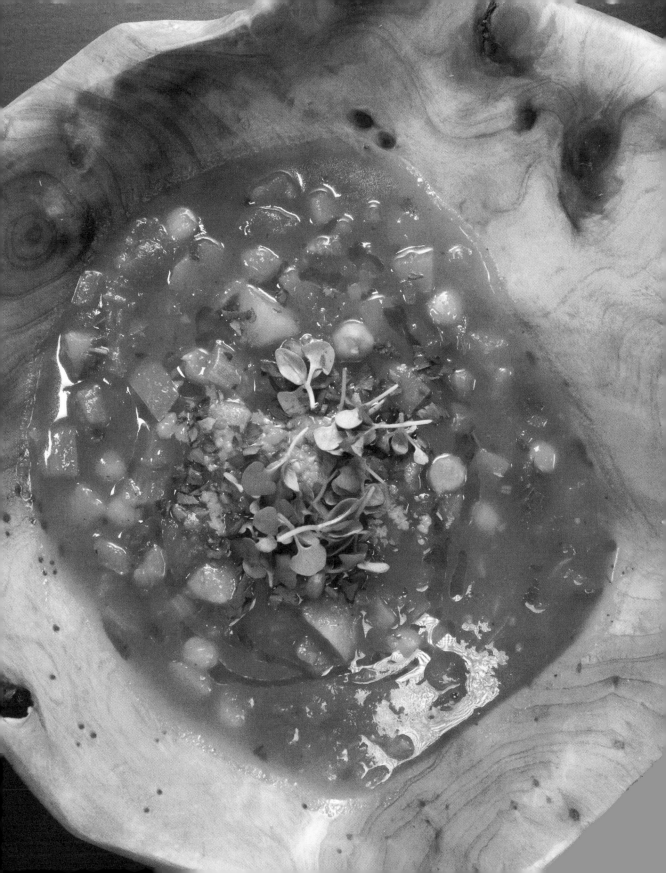

RAINBOW & SUNSHINE BOWL

SERVES 2   PREP TIME 15 MIN   COOKING TIME 23 TO 30 MIN   TOTAL TIME 38 TO 45 MIN

This bowl is an absolute powerhouse! If you're looking to lose a little weight, or just eat something a little healthier, this recipe is stacked high with protein, fiber, iron, antioxidants, and essential vitamins. And just look at those colors! I don't know about you, but sometimes, after a weekend of partying or a phase of eating out, all I want to do is cleanse my body. And unlike my friend who swears by juicing (you know who you are)—which, by the way, meant something very different back in the '90s—I like to eat super-clean, fiber-rich foods that will help clean everything out of my gut and intestinal tract. This dish does exactly that—plus, it's low-calorie and high in protein. So the next time you feel like you want some good-tasting fiber in your diet, this bowl is the one!

Sea salt

1 sweet potato (about 12 ounces), peeled and cubed

1 tablespoon olive oil

Freshly ground black pepper

1 cup fresh or frozen shelled edamame

1 cup fresh or frozen corn kernels

1 cup shredded red cabbage

2 cups coarsely chopped curly kale (leaves only)

1 small carrot, thinly shredded

1 small beet, peeled and thinly shredded

1/4 cup Tahini Vinaigrette (recipe follows)

1 teaspoon toasted sesame seeds, for garnish

1. Preheat the oven to 425°F. Bring a medium pot of salted water to a boil.

2. On a rimmed baking sheet, toss the sweet potatoes with the olive oil and season with salt and pepper. Roast until tender and browned in spots, 20 to 25 minutes, flipping once halfway through the cooking time.

3. Meanwhile, add the edamame to the boiling water and cook until tender, 2 to 3 minutes. Using a slotted spoon or handheld strainer, transfer the edamame to a plate. Bring the water back to a boil and add the corn; cook until tender, 1 to 2 minutes. Drain the corn and transfer it to the plate with the edamame (keeping them separate on the plate).

4. Divide the roasted sweet potatoes, edamame, corn, cabbage, kale, carrot, and beet between two shallow bowls. Drizzle the tahini vinaigrette over the top. Garnish with the sesame seeds and serve.

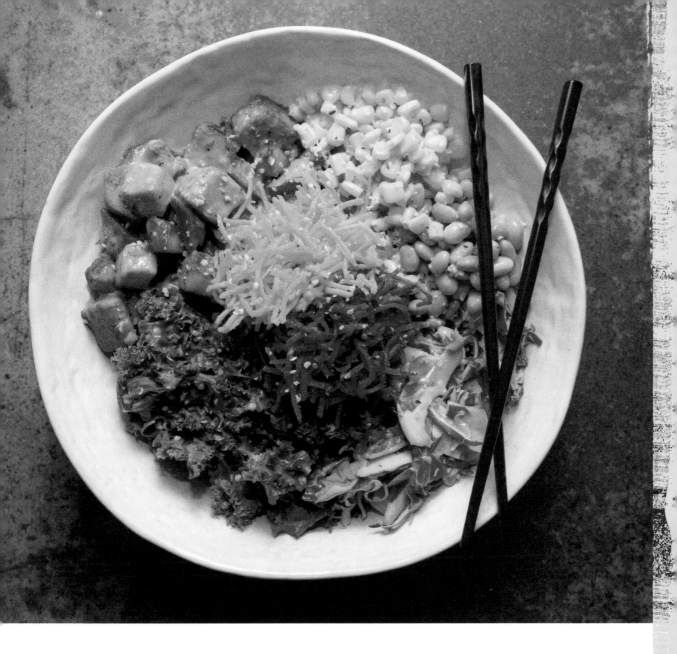

TAHINI VINAIGRETTE

MAKES ½ CUP

2 tablespoons tahini

¼ cup olive oil

¼ cup apple cider vinegar

1 teaspoon agave or pure
  maple syrup

Sea salt and freshly ground
  black pepper

In a glass mason jar, combine the tahini, oil, vinegar, and agave. Seal the jar and shake until well blended. Season with salt and pepper. Store in the refrigerator for up to 1 week.

ONLY-PLANTS-ALLOWED BURGER

SERVES 4   PREP TIME 20 MIN   COOKING TIME 35 MIN   TOTAL TIME 55 MIN

I love imitation "beef" burgers as much as the next guy, but sometimes I do crave a real veggie burger, you know? Remember growing up, when a veggie burger actually meant a burger made from vegetables? Yeah, that thing. As amazing as it is that all the fast-food chains are starting to introduce meat alternatives on their menus, we're losing sight of what it actually means to eat whole foods. I never thought I would have this problem, but sometimes it's really difficult finding a good veggie burger made from actual vegetables. But like anything I have trouble finding—I just create it! So the next time you're having a barbecue or just want a patty made from real veggies, give this recipe a shot. Serve it on your favorite bun with your go-to toppings, and I promise you'll feel better about your health and your food!

2 tablespoons flaxseed meal

6 ounces white button mushrooms, quartered

1 medium carrot, cut into ½-inch pieces

½ pound broccoli crowns, cut into ½-inch florets

1 small yellow onion, quartered

2 garlic cloves, smashed

5 to 6 tablespoons avocado oil

1 teaspoon paprika

1 teaspoon chili powder

Sea salt and freshly ground black pepper

1 (15-ounce) can black beans, drained and rinsed

⅓ cup walnuts

2 cups packed baby spinach

Leaves from ½ small bunch parsley

1 small bunch chives, coarsely chopped

½ cup gluten-free bread crumbs

1 tablespoon tomato paste

¾ cup cooked brown rice

4 burger buns

Toppings of your choice

1   Preheat the oven to 400°F. Line a rimmed baking sheet with parchment paper.

2   In a small bowl, whisk the flaxseed meal with 5 tablespoons water and refrigerate to thicken while you proceed with the recipe (this mixture will be your "flax eggs").

3   In a food processor, combine the mushrooms, carrot, broccoli, onion, garlic, 2 tablespoons of the oil, the paprika, and the chili powder. Season with salt and pepper. Pulse until coarsely chopped. Spread the vegetable mixture in an even layer over the prepared baking sheet. Bake for 15 minutes.

4   Stir the vegetables, then push them to one side of the baking sheet. On the other side of the sheet, toss the black beans with 1 tablespoon of the oil, then spread them into an even layer. Bake until the vegetables are tender and the black beans are dried a bit (you want some of the moisture to evaporate, but they should still be soft when pinched), about 10 minutes. Remove from the oven and let cool for 10 minutes.

5   Rinse and dry the food processor bowl and blade. Place the walnuts, spinach, parsley, chives and 1 tablespoon of the oil in the food processor. Pulse to a pestolike consistency.

6   Add the black beans to the food processor and pulse a few times, until the beans are broken down a little. Add the vegetable mixture, the bread crumbs, tomato paste, and flax eggs. Pulse until mixed (the mixture should have a coarse texture).

7   Scrape the mixture into a large bowl. Add the rice and, using a fork, stir to combine (the mixture will be thick, but it will come together). Form the vegetable-rice mixture into eight 4-inch patties.

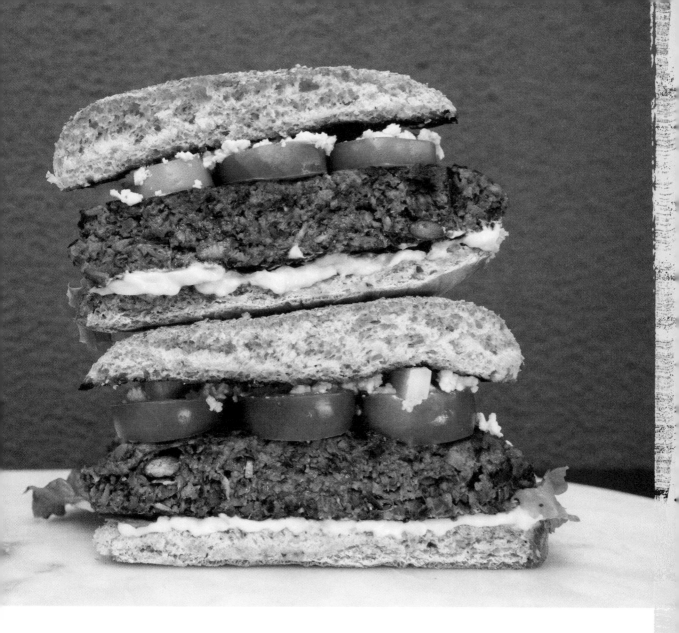

8　In a large nonstick skillet, heat 1 tablespoon of the oil over medium heat. Add half the patties and cook, flipping once, until browned on both sides, about 5 minutes per side. Repeat with the remaining patties, adding 1 tablespoon more oil to the pan between batches, if needed.

9　Put the patties on buns and serve with your favorite toppings.

TIP

Don't flip the burger until it is golden brown on one side, or it may fall apart. Alternatively, after you form the patties, put them in the freezer for 10 minutes to help them set and hold together, then cook them.

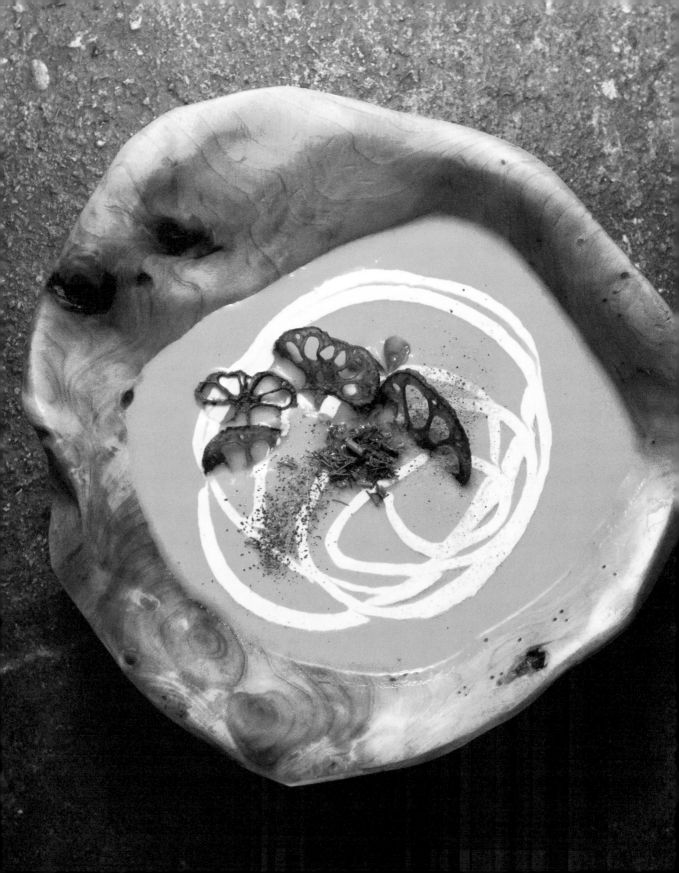

From Indigo Age Cafe in Vancouver, Canada

BUTTERNUT SQUASH SOUP

SERVES 4   PREP TIME 10 MIN, PLUS 5 MIN COOLING
COOKING TIME 20 MIN   TOTAL TIME 30 TO 35 MIN

I visited Indigo Age Cafe during the autumn season when they had beautiful squashes, root vegetables, and cranberries in house, so naturally I was drawn to some of their recipes that were appropriate for Thanksgiving. Nothing says "plant-based Thanksgiving" more than this recipe right here. It's warm, comforting, creamy, and pretty simple to make, which means you don't have to slave away preparing a Thanksgiving dinner for your guests. Who needs turkey?! It just takes away hours of time you could be spending with your friends and family. And the best thing about this recipe is that you can use any squash you have available to you. Indigo recommends banana squash, kabocha squash, or pumpkin if you can't get butternut. This holiday season, squash your kitchen time in half and spend some more time with your loved ones! Get it? Butternut squash soup, squash your kitchen time . . . oh, never mind!

2 teaspoons avocado oil
   or other neutral oil

1 shallot, finely chopped

1 garlic clove, finely chopped

1 pound peeled, cubed
   butternut squash

1 celery stalk, finely chopped

1 carrot, finely chopped

1 tablespoon finely chopped
   fresh flat-leaf parsley

Dash of ground cinnamon

Dash of ground nutmeg

Dash of ground cloves

Sea salt and freshly ground
   black pepper

1 teaspoon finely chopped
   fresh dill

FOR THE CREAMY CASHEW DRIZZLE

1 cup raw cashews, soaked in
   water to cover for 2 hours
   and drained

1 garlic clove

1 tablespoon freshly squeezed
   lemon juice

1 tablespoon nutritional yeast

Pinch of sea salt

1 teaspoon finely chopped
   fresh dill, for garnish

1 In a heavy-bottomed medium pot, heat the oil over medium heat. Add the shallot and garlic. Cook, stirring occasionally, until the shallot is softened, about 3 minutes.

2 Add the squash, celery, carrot, parsley, cinnamon, nutmeg, and cloves; season with salt and pepper. Add 2 cups water and bring to a boil, then reduce the heat to medium-low and simmer until the squash is very tender, 15 to 20 minutes. Remove from the heat and let cool for 5 minutes.

3 Meanwhile, make the creamy cashew drizzle: In a blender, combine the cashews, garlic, lemon juice, nutritional yeast, salt, and 3/4 cup water. Blend until smooth. Transfer to a bowl.

4 Rinse the blender jar. Working in batches, carefully ladle the soup (broth and vegetables) into the blender. Cover the blender jar, place a towel over the lid, and blend until smooth (be careful of splatter, as soup will still be hot).

5 Pour the pureed soup into four deep serving bowls; repeat to puree the remaining soup. Swirl some of the creamy cashew drizzle in each bowl. Sprinkle with pepper, garnish with the dill, and serve.

TIP

For an extra-special treat, dehydrate your own lotus root for garnish: Cut the lotus root crosswise into very thin slices and place them on a baking sheet. Coat with oil and season with freshly ground black pepper, sea salt, and paprika. Bake at 325°F for 45 minutes until crisp, flipping the slices once halfway through.

CHICK'N SALAD

SERVES 4   PREP TIME 30 MIN   COOKING TIME 25 MIN   TOTAL TIME 55 MIN

I don't know about you, but I always underestimate salad. Salad is like that person you went out with one time on a very awkward date and then see across the street months later—you make sure you avoid eye contact at all costs. I was the same way when we first walked into The Sudra in Portland. When the chef brought out this dish, I thought, *Really, dude, you're having us try the salad at an Indian restaurant?* But boy oh boy, was I glad he brought this heavenly creation out of that kitchen. Loaded with kale, corn, beets, and yam, this salad is not only oozing with vitamins and minerals, but there's a lot of flavor intricately layered into this dish. So the next time you want a recipe that will make your friends believers in the power of salad, start chopping up that kale. All hail the kale!

FOR THE ROASTED ROOT VEGETABLES

- 1 pound beets, peeled and diced
- 1 pound sweet potatoes, diced
- 3 carrots, diced
- 3 tablespoons olive oil
- 1 teaspoon sea salt
- Freshly ground black pepper

FOR THE CHICK'N

- 1 (8-ounce) package vegan chick'n strips
- 3 cups boiling water
- 1½ tablespoons olive oil
- ½ red bell pepper, finely chopped
- ½ small yellow onion, finely chopped
- ¼ cup fresh or frozen corn kernels

- 2 garlic cloves, minced
- 1 teaspoon minced fresh ginger
- 1 teaspoon paprika
- 1 teaspoon ground coriander
- 1 teaspoon chili powder

FOR THE DRESSING

- 1 tablespoon olive oil
- 1 tablespoon tahini
- 1 tablespoon white wine or apple cider vinegar
- Sea salt and freshly ground black pepper

- 1 cup packed coarsely chopped curly kale leaves

1. Preheat the oven to 450°F.

2. On a rimmed baking sheet, toss the beets, sweet potatoes, carrots, and olive oil and season with the salt and pepper to taste. Bake until tender, 15 to 20 minutes.

3. Meanwhile, prepare the chick'n: In a medium bowl, combine the vegan strips and boiling water; set aside to soften for 10 to 15 minutes, then drain.

4. In a large skillet, heat the olive oil over medium-high heat. Add the bell pepper, onion, and corn. Cook until softened and browned in spots, 3 to 4 minutes. Add the garlic and ginger and cook until fragrant, about 1 minute. Add the paprika, coriander, and chili powder and stir to coat. Stir in 2 tablespoons water and remove from the heat.

5. Make the dressing: In a large bowl, whisk together the olive oil, tahini, and vinegar and season with salt and pepper.

6. Add the kale to the bowl with the dressing and toss to combine. Divide the kale among individual serving dishes. Add the roasted root vegetables to the skillet with the vegan strips, stir to combine, then spoon the mixture over the kale and serve.

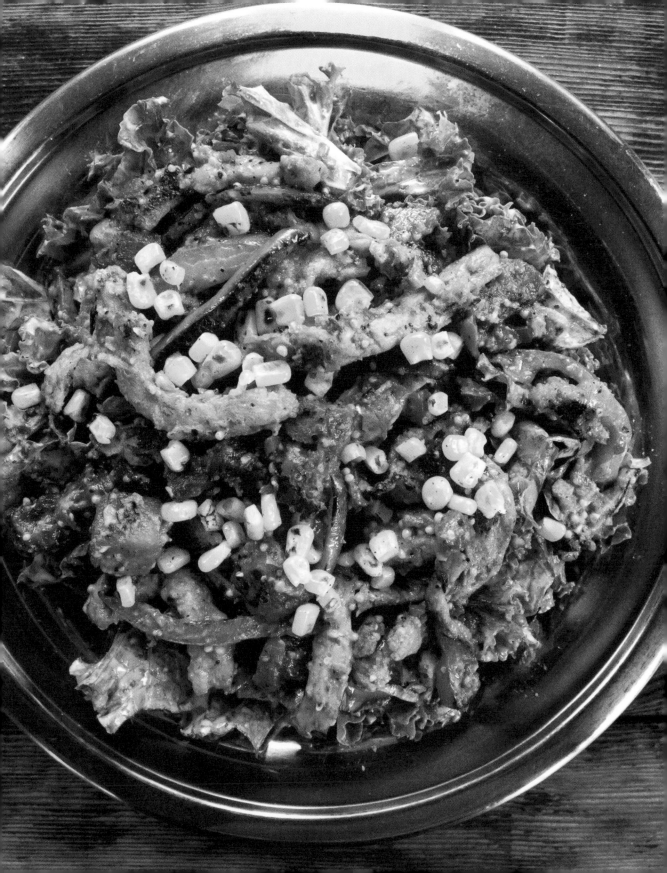

CHICK'N SCHNITZEL

SERVES 6   **PREP TIME** 40 MIN   **COOKING TIME** 5 MIN   **TOTAL TIME** 45 MIN

When I first transitioned to a plant-based diet, it was hard to imagine that I would ever eat a warm, breaded, topped-with-the-perfect-tomato-sauce schnitzel ever again. But thanks to the growing vegan culinary community, now I can have all the schnitzel I want, without any of the cholesterol! Breaded-and-fried anything is never going to be "healthy," but the elimination of cholesterol definitely makes me feel better about eating this dish. Now, this recipe isn't the easiest because it requires you to make your own vegan chicken from scratch (but this recipe is also quite difficult to get your hands on, so thank you to YamChops for sharing!). Having said that, if you're running tight on time or just don't feel like dealing with vital wheat gluten, you can buy prepared chick'n cutlets, and follow this recipe for the breading, tomato sauce, and delicious sautéed veggies. Or use vegan chicken nuggets for little bite-size schnitzels that will impress the heck out of your guests!

1 (15-ounce) can chickpeas, drained and rinsed

3 tablespoons olive oil

3 tablespoons tamari

1 tablespoon tahini

2 teaspoons Hungarian paprika

2 teaspoons dried thyme

1 teaspoon garlic powder

1 cup vital wheat gluten

1 ¾ cups plain bread crumbs, plus more if needed

4 tablespoons egg replacer

½ cup vegetable broth

2 tablespoons grapeseed oil, plus more for frying

1 medium yellow onion, thinly sliced

Sea salt

8 ounces cremini (baby bella) mushrooms, thinly sliced

All-purpose flour, for dusting

6 kaiser rolls

¼ cup jarred marinara sauce, warmed, for serving

1   In a food processor, combine the chickpeas, olive oil, tamari, tahini, paprika, thyme, and garlic powder and pulse a few times just to coarsely chop the chickpeas. Scrape down the sides of the bowl.

2   Add the vital wheat gluten, 1 cup of the bread crumbs, and 2 tablespoons of the egg replacer; pulse again to combine (the mixture will be a bit dry). With the food processor running, drizzle in the broth (you may not need it all) until the mixture comes together to form a firm dough; it should be tacky but not wet or sticky.

3   Transfer the dough to a cutting board or the counter and form it into a ball. If it's too wet or sticky, knead in more bread crumbs 1 tablespoon at a time until the dough is just tacky. Cover the dough loosely with a clean kitchen towel and let rest for 30 minutes.

4   Meanwhile, in a large nonstick skillet, heat 1 tablespoon of the grapeseed oil over medium-high heat. Add the onion, season with salt, and cook until softened and barely golden, about 2 minutes. Transfer to a plate.

5   In the same skillet, heat the remaining 1 tablespoon grapeseed oil over medium-high heat. Add the mushrooms and cook, stirring occasionally, until softened and golden, about 2 minutes. Transfer the mushrooms to the plate with the onion.

6   Fill the same skillet with ¼ inch of grapeseed oil and heat the oil over medium-high heat. Line a plate with a paper towel and set it nearby.

7   In a shallow bowl, whisk together the remaining 2 tablespoons egg replacer and ¼ cup water. Put the remaining ¾ cup bread crumbs in a separate shallow bowl and season with salt.

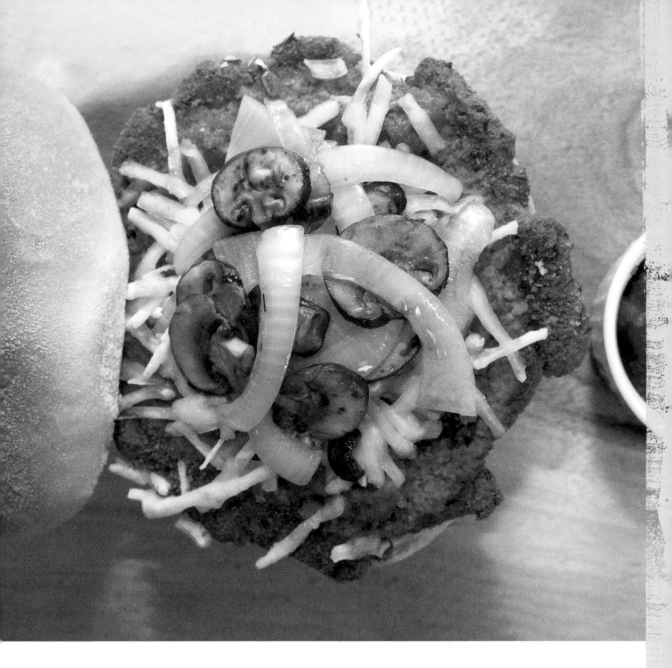

8   Lightly flour a cutting board or the counter. Divide the dough into 6 even pieces and roll
them into balls. Roll each ball of dough out to 1/4 inch thick, then dust the "cutlet" with flour.
Working with one at a time, dip the "cutlets" into the egg replacer, letting any excess drip off,
then dip them in the bread crumbs, turning once to coat completely, and shake off any excess.

9   Add the cutlets to the hot oil, a few at a time so as to not crowd the pan, and cook, flipping
once, until browned on both sides, 1 to 2 minutes per side. Transfer to the prepared plate to
drain and repeat with the remaining cutlets.

10 Put a cutlet on each roll, top with some of the marinara sauce and sautéed onions and
mushrooms, and serve.

PHILLY CHEESESTEAK

SERVES 2   PREP TIME 5 MIN   COOKING TIME 7 TO 10 MIN   TOTAL TIME 12 TO 15 MIN

The truth is, nothing with the name "Philly cheesesteak" is healthy. Not even the vegan version. So if you're looking for a healthy sandwich (and there's a lot of them in this book), just go right ahead and turn the page, because, Mamma, this is one to indulge in. I distinctly remember this sandwich from our tour because I cooked it myself . . . while the owner of Mission Square Market, Sonny, was yelling instructions at me from across the kitchen—"STIR IN THE CHEESE, STIR IN THE CHEESE!" Truth be told, he was the kindest man we met on the whole tour, but, boy, was he passionate about vegan cheese. Needless to say, I never forget to stir in the cheese in this recipe, and neither should you.

- 2 (8-inch) Italian hero rolls, split in half
- 1 ½ tablespoons safflower oil, plus more for drizzling
- 15 slices vegan roast beef (about one 5.5-ounce package Tofurky roast beef)
- 1 green bell pepper, thinly spiced
- 1 medium yellow onion, thinly sliced
- Sea salt and freshly ground black pepper
- 5 slices vegan provolone cheese
- 1 tablespoon vegan mayonnaise (optional)

1. Heat a medium skillet over medium-high heat. Drizzle the cut sides of the rolls with oil and place them in the pan, cut-side down. Cook until toasted, 1 to 2 minutes. Transfer to a cutting board.

2. In the same skillet, heat ½ tablespoon of the oil over medium-high heat. Working in batches, add the vegan roast beef and cook until heated and lightly browned, 1 to 2 minutes per side. Transfer to the cutting board with bread.

3. Add the remaining 1 tablespoon oil to the skillet and heat over medium-high heat. Add the bell pepper and onion and season with salt and black pepper. Cook until the onion is softened and the bell pepper is tender, 5 to 6 minutes, adding water 1 tablespoon at a time as needed if the pan gets too dry.

4. Return the roast beef to the pan with all of your other ingredients, top with the cheese, cover, and cook until the cheese has melted, about 2 minutes.

5. Spread the mayo (if using) over the toasted sides of the rolls. Pile the peppers, onions, and roast beef with melted provolone onto the bottom halves of the rolls, cover with the top halves, and serve immediately.

TOASTED JACKFRUIT TUNA SANDWICH

SERVES 2 **PREP TIME** 10 MIN **COOKING TIME** 4 MIN **TOTAL TIME** ABOUT 15 MIN

We all have our own tuna sandwich story. Whether you were embarrassed when you brought it to school that one time, or couldn't kiss your high school crush because of your tuna breath (even though you had a perfect moment), or you and your mother had a screaming match in the kitchen because you disagreed on the merits of it, we all have a story to share about this infamous, smelly, but undeniably delicious sandwich. My mom used to feed us tuna fish all the time because it is laughably easy to make, incredibly cheap, and very filling. Needless to say, when I discovered this timeless classic *veganized* at Off The Griddle, all I could hope for was that it tasted as good as my mom's. And I have to tell you, jackfruit is a genius substitute! Once it's flaked, it looks exactly like tuna, and it naturally absorbs a ton of flavor! So give this recipe a try or even make it the way your mom used to make her tuna sandwiches, and I promise you will not be disappointed. Pair it with your favorite chips, and you'll truly be turning back time.

1 (14-ounce) can jackfruit
   (preferably Native Forest),
   drained

1 cup vegan mayonnaise,
   plus more for serving

1 tablespoon mustard powder

1 teaspoon dulse flakes

1½ teaspoons onion powder

1½ teaspoons garlic powder

1 teaspoons paprika

1 tablespoon freshly squeezed
   lemon juice

2 tablespoons nutritional
   yeast

2 tablespoons agave syrup

Sea salt and freshly ground
   black pepper

1½ tablespoons vegan butter

4 slices bread

1 or 2 slices vegan cheese
   of your choice (optional)

Toppings of your choice,
   such as lettuce and tomato

1. Put the jackfruit in a medium bowl and use a fork to shred it into a tuna-like consistency.

2. In a blender, combine the mayonnaise, mustard powder, dulse flakes, onion powder, garlic powder, paprika, lemon juice, nutritional yeast, and agave syrup. Blend until smooth and transfer to the bowl with the jackfruit. Season with salt and pepper and gently fold to combine.

3. In a large skillet, melt the butter over medium-high heat. Add the bread and cook, flipping once, until toasted, about 2 minutes per side. (If using the cheese, add it after flipping the bread and allow it to melt.)

4. Place a slice of toasted bread on each of two plates. Divide the tuna between them and add toppings, as desired. Top with the remaining bread and serve immediately.

FUN FACT

Believe it or not, they make canned vegan tuna now, so feel free to use that instead of jackfruit if you ever see it at your local grocer!

MAGICAL MANGO CURRY WRAP

SERVES 1   PREP TIME 20 MIN   TOTAL TIME 20 MIN

The one fruit that reminds me most of Egypt has to be the mango. We left Egypt to immigrate to Canada when I was three years old, but whenever we went back to visit, I remember being blown away by how different the mangoes tasted there. Even recently, on a trip to Egypt with my sisters and parents, I could not believe how much sweeter, thicker, and juicier the mangoes were! Needless to say, mangoes are one of my favorite fruits on the planet. That's why I love this wrap from Peace Pies, filled with whole foods (and mango) in a coconut tortilla, with a side of . . . you guessed it: mango curry sauce. If you want something light and truly refreshing for lunch, this is a winner! And if you like mango . . . what the heck are you waiting for?

1 Coconut Curry Coco-tilla
(recipe follows) or store-
bought coconut wrap
(see Tip)

1 collard green leaf, stemmed

1 cup sprouts

3 thick mango slices

3 thick avocado slices

¼ cup shredded purple
cabbage

¼ cup shredded carrots

Handful of fresh greens

Coconut Curry Sauce
(recipe follows)

1 On the bottom half of the coconut wrap, layer the collard leaf, sprouts, mango, avocado, cabbage, carrots, and greens. Drizzle with sauce.

2 Roll up the wrap like a burrito to enclose the filling and cut it in half. Serve with some extra sauce on the side, if desired.

TIP

If you prefer not to make your own, you can find coconut wraps at Whole Foods or online from sources like Thrive Market.

COCONUT CURRY COCO-TILLA

MAKES 4

4 cups chopped fresh coconut
meat

1 teaspoon sesame oil

⅓ cup agave syrup or
coconut nectar

¼ cup freshly squeezed
lemon juice

1 ½ tablespoons curry powder

½ teaspoon sea salt

1 cup coconut water

1 Combine the coconut meat, oil, agave syrup, lemon juice, curry powder, salt, and coconut water in a blender and puree until smooth.

2 Scoop 1 cup of the mixture onto a dehydrator sheet and spread it evenly into a 10-inch round. Repeat with the remaining mixture, using a separate dehydrator sheet for each round. Dehydrate overnight at 105°F. You can store this in the referigrator for up to 3 days.

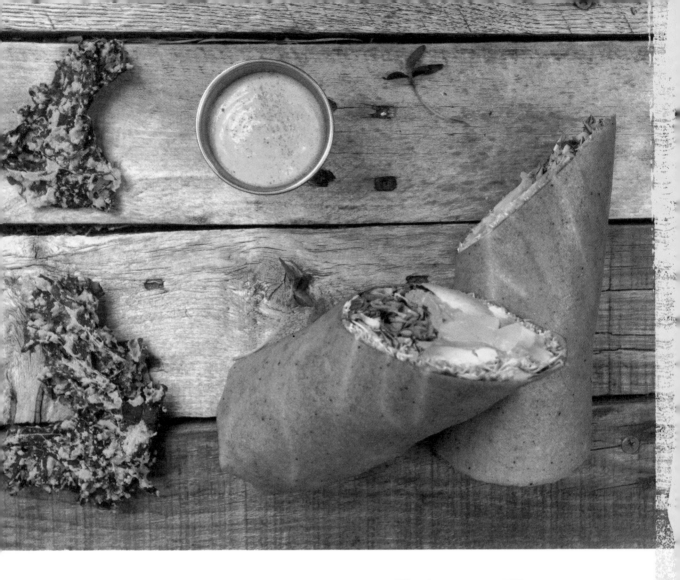

COCONUT CURRY SAUCE

SERVES 2 TO 4

1 ½ cups chopped young
   coconut meat

3 tablespoons freshly
   squeezed lemon juice

1 tablespoon curry powder

½ cup coconut water

1 teaspoon sea salt

1 teaspoon ground coriander

1 teaspoon garlic powder
   (optional)

1 teaspoon onion powder
   (optional)

Combine the coconut meat, lemon juice, curry powder, coconut water, salt, coriander, and, if using, the garlic powder and onion powder in a blender and puree until smooth. Store in an airtight container for up to 5 days.

BBQ PULLED "PORK" JACKFRUIT SANDWICH

SERVES 2   **PREP TIME** 10 MIN   **COOKING TIME** 1 HR   **TOTAL TIME** 1 HR 10 MIN

Jackfruit is another one of those foods that has come out of nowhere. And if you've never seen the actual fruit, please search for it! (I always argue with people because I think it looks like a green koala bear and no one ever agrees.) If you've ever cooked with jackfruit, you know that it soaks up flavor like a desperate sponge and has an incredibly meaty texture, which is why people love using it for tacos, bowls, and, in this case, sandwiches. Pulled pork sandwiches, to be exact! So the next time you're in the mood for BBQ without having to actually barbecue, this recipe is going to satisfy your cravings and maybe start a heated debate about how exotic fruits can look like cute little animals!

FOR THE BBQ JACKFRUIT

- 1 small yellow onion, finely chopped
- 2 garlic cloves, finely chopped
- 1 apple, peeled, cored, and finely chopped
- 1/2 cup barbecue sauce
- 1/4 cup soy sauce
- 1 tablespoon sesame oil
- 1 tablespoon Dijon mustard
- 1/4 teaspoon sea salt
- 1 (20-ounce) can jackfruit, drained

FOR THE SAUTÉED ONION

- 1 tablespoon neutral oil, such as grapeseed or safflower
- 1 medium yellow onion, thinly sliced
- Sea salt and freshly ground black pepper

FOR THE SLAW

- 1 1/2 teaspoons apple cider vinegar
- 1 1/2 teaspoons neutral oil, such as grapeseed or safflower
- Sea salt and freshly ground black pepper
- 1 cup shredded coleslaw blend

- 2 kaiser or hero rolls, split lengthwise and toasted

1 Make the BBQ jackfruit: In a medium pot, combine the onion, garlic, apple, barbecue sauce, soy sauce, sesame oil, mustard, salt, and 1/2 cup water. Bring to a boil over medium-high heat.

2 Add the jackfruit, reduce the heat to low, and simmer until the sauce has reduced and thickened and the jackfruit easily falls apart when smashed with a fork, about 45 minutes.

3 Meanwhile, sauté the onion: In a medium skillet, heat the oil over medium heat. Add the onion and season with salt and pepper. Cook, stirring occasionally, until tender and browned, about 5 minutes. Set aside.

4 Make the slaw: In a medium bowl, whisk together the vinegar and oil; season with salt and pepper. Add the coleslaw blend and toss to combine. Chill or set aside at room temperature until ready to serve.

5 To finish the jackfruit, increase the heat under the pot to medium-high. Cook until the jackfruit gets crispy in spots and the sauce clings to it, 2 to 3 minutes.

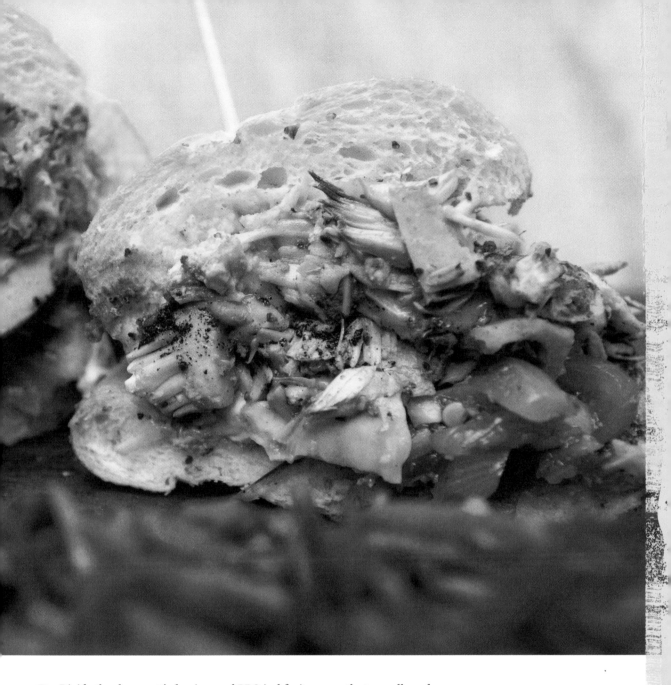

6   Divide the slaw, sautéed onion, and BBQ jackfruit among the two rolls and serve.

TIP

For the coleslaw, any creamy or vinaigrette
dressing you have or want to purchase
works fine here. You're primarily looking
to add some crunch to your sandwich to
balance out the soft texture of the BBQ
jackfruit and sautéed onion.

TOFU POMEGRANATE SALAD

SERVES 2 TO 4   **PREP TIME** 10 MIN   **COOKING TIME** 15 MIN   **TOTAL TIME** 25 MIN

A lot of people stress out about not getting enough iron, B12, or omegas in their plant-based diets, and that is a completely valid concern. But what I find myself lacking most often in my diet is a healthy and nutritious salad. Salads are a great way to add many of those vitamins and minerals you feel like you aren't getting enough of. And while the vegan Caesar salad is becoming the new hype around town, it doesn't satiate my need for something light, crisp, and nutritious. The added bonus of this recipe is that you can make extras of all the components and save them in your fridge for other dishes. The green goddess dressing and blackened tofu can be used on a plethora of other salads, sandwiches, and bowls, and the sunflower seeds make for a very satisfying snack all on their own. And because this dish screams "summer" to me, I'd recommend serving it on a hot, sunny, summer day, before a BBQ or by the pool! Whatever the occasion, this salad is a crowd-pleaser.

1 (14-ounce) package extra-firm tofu, thoroughly drained

1 to 2 teaspoons Cajun seasoning, depending on taste

½ cup sunflower seeds

1 tablespoon sesame oil

6 cups mesclun salad mix

½ cup Green Goddess Dressing (recipe follows)

1 pear, cored and thinly sliced, for serving

½ cup fresh pomegranate seeds, for garnish

1   Evenly cut the tofu lengthwise into 4 pieces, then halve each piece diagonally into triangles. Season the tofu all over with the Cajun seasoning and set aside.

2   Heat a medium nonstick skillet over medium-high heat. Add the sunflower seeds and cook, shaking the pan, until fragrant and lightly toasted, about 3 minutes. Transfer to a plate to cool.

3   In the same skillet, heat the sesame oil over medium-high heat. Working in batches, add the tofu and cook, turning once, until golden and crisp on both sides, 2 to 3 minutes per side. Transfer to a paper towel–lined plate.

4   In a large bowl, toss the mesclun mix and dressing until well coated. Divide the dressed salad among individual serving plates. Top with the tofu and pear slices. Sprinkle the pomegranate seeds and toasted sunflower seeds over the top. Serve immediately.

TIP

In order to prevent the mesclun mix from turning soggy, do not toss it with the dressing until you are ready to serve.

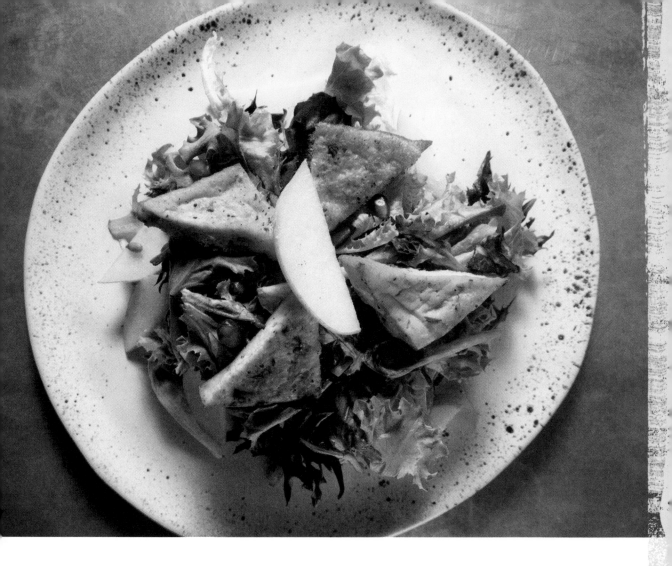

GREEN GODDESS DRESSING

MAKES ABOUT 1 ½ CUPS

1 garlic clove, smashed and
   peeled

1 cup vegan mayonnaise

½ cup tahini

½ cup fresh flat-leaf parsley
   leaves

¼ cup fresh tarragon leaves

2 scallions, finely chopped

2 tablespoons freshly
   squeezed lemon juice

Sea salt

Combine the garlic, mayonnaise, tahini, parsley, tarragon, scallions,
and lemon juice in a blender. Blend until smooth. Season with salt.
Store in an airtight container in the refrigerator for up to 1 week.

SAN FRANCI

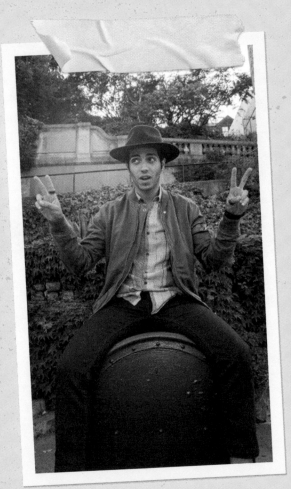

I HAD BEEN LOOKING FORWARD TO VISITING SAN FRANCISCO FOR A VERY LONG TIME, MAYBE FOR NO OTHER REASON THAN TO VISIT THE CITY WHERE ONE OF MY FAVORITE FILMS OF ALL TIME WAS FILMED: *MRS. DOUBTFIRE.*

Not only that, but it was actually Robin Williams's favorite place to live, and his ashes were scattered along the San Francisco Bay. And I can tell why Robin liked it so much. It's a very eclectic place, where the very rich and the very poor live alongside each other. There's immense wealth in San Francisco but also a gritty culture and grind that makes it feel alive, much like New York City.

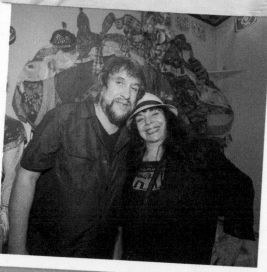

SCO

And that's also true about the food scene. There are places like WeTheTrillions, which feels very modern, new, and health-focused, and places like Peña Pachamama that have existed for over twenty years without changing. When you walk into Peña Pachamama, you feel like you are transported back to the '80s (and, in fact, it was one of the spots Robin Williams frequented).

The plant-based scene in San Francisco has everything from modern vegan fare to authentic Bolivian food. With an incredible local culture and nightlife, San Fran has it all, and if you're looking for some incredibly varied and beautiful plant-based food, you'll have a whole list of places to check out the next time you're there. So, in the words of one of Hollywood's and San Francisco's legends, I will leave you with this: "Yo! I'm a raptor, doin' what I can, gonna eat everything till the appearance of man. Yo, yo, see me, I'm livin' below the soil, I'll be back but I'm comin' as oil!"

QUENTIN & EDDY NAVIA
Owners, Peña Pachamama

The restaurant industry is tough! It's a hell of a lot of work opening a restaurant, and even more difficult sustaining one—let alone for twenty years! The hallowed space that now holds Peña Pachamama has a long history of entertainment, from its time as one of the most popular speakeasies in all of San Francisco to when it was converted to Amelio's, which hosted celebrities like Dean Martin, Rocky Marciano, and even President Kennedy. When Quentin Navia took over the space, she wanted to honor that history and build on those traditions. And so, Peña Pachamama, a plant-based Bolivian restaurant/bar with live Latin music and performances, was born!

When you first walk into this space, you can feel the history of it. The wallpaper looks like the original art deco, the walls are lined with black-and-white photos of famous celebrities, and the stage—yes, the stage—is one that you can imagine the likes of Frank Sinatra or Miles Davis performing on during dinner service back in the '50s or '60s. Needless to say, Peña Pachamama exudes a deep culture of food and music—the two pillars Quentin and her husband, Eddy, have built this place on. And unlike any of the other restaurants we visited in San Francisco, this one doesn't try to be modern or hip. It serves unique, delicious Bolivian food and stands firm in its history. More than just a vegan restaurant or bar, it's a historical monument in the heart of San Fran. So the next time you're visiting the Golden City, make sure you peek your head into Peña Pachamama and say hello to Quentin and Eddy!

CHAPTER 4

ENTRÉES

Featuring recipes from or inspired by:

AVIV
PORTLAND, OREGON

BUNNA CAFE
BROOKLYN, NEW YORK

DONNA JEAN
SAN DIEGO, CALIFORNIA

FANCY RADISH
WASHINGTON, DC

HEIRLOOM
VANCOUVER, CANADA

ICHIZA KITCHEN
PORTLAND, OREGON

MAMMA'S KITCHEN

MY HOME KITCHEN

PLANTA YORKVILLE
TORONTO, CANADA

THE SUDRA
PORTLAND, OREGON

TACO PARTY
BOSTON, MASSACHUSETTS

VIRTUOUS PIE
VANCOUVER, CANADA

WETHETRILLIONS
SAN FRANCISCO, CALIFORNIA

YAMCHOPS
TORONTO, CANADA

ADOBE-FERMENTED SOY CHICKEN

SERVES **2 TO 4**   PREP TIME **20 MIN, PLUS OVERNIGHT MARINATING**
COOKING TIME **35 MIN**   TOTAL TIME **55 MIN**

It's not often I go to a restaurant and experience something completely original. And from our whole tour, I have to say this dish from Ichiza was the most unique food I tried on our whole tour. The only other time my palate has ever felt this sense of wonderment was when I visited Japan, but that's a story for another day. This Adobe-Fermented Soy Chicken was so unlike anything I have ever tried, and I am incredibly grateful Cyrus, the chef-owner of Ichiza Kitchen, agreed to contribute the recipe for this book. The use of earthy ingredients like bay leaves and garlic combined with the acid from the coconut vinegar and soy sauce is outstanding. And all that savory chicken combined with onions, carrots, and rice is a match made in heaven! I think about this dish and all the dishes at Ichiza often, so if you are ever in Portland, make sure you check out Cyrus's culinary adventure.

2 cups vegetable broth

$\frac{1}{2}$ cup plus $\frac{1}{2}$ teaspoon soy sauce

$\frac{1}{4}$ cup white wine vinegar

1 large yellow onion, chopped into 1-inch pieces

1 garlic clove, finely chopped

1 bay leaf, preferably fresh, but dried is okay

$\frac{1}{2}$ teaspoon freshly ground black pepper, plus more if needed

1 pound vegan soy chicken or seitan, shredded or crumbled into large pieces

2 carrots, thinly sliced on an angle

2 tablespoons neutral oil, such as grapeseed or safflower

$\frac{1}{2}$ pint grape tomatoes

2 teaspoons freshly squeezed lemon juice

2 cups cooked jasmine or sushi rice, for serving

1. In a large bowl, combine the broth, $\frac{1}{2}$ cup of the soy sauce, the vinegar, onion, garlic, bay leaf, and pepper. Add the soy chicken and carrots, toss to combine, then cover and marinate in the refrigerator overnight or for at least 8 hours.

2. Place a fine-mesh sieve over a bowl. Drain the soy chicken and vegetables, reserving the marinade.

3. In a medium pot, heat the oil over medium-high heat until very hot. Add the soy chicken and vegetables (the oil may splatter, so be careful). Cook, stirring occasionally, until golden brown in spots, about 3 minutes.

4. Add the reserved marinade to the pot. Bring to a boil, then reduce the heat to medium-low. Taste and season with more pepper, if needed. Simmer until the vegetables are tender and the marinade has reduced by half, 20 to 25 minutes; season to taste with salt, if needed.

5. Meanwhile, in a medium bowl, combine the tomatoes, lemon juice, and remaining $\frac{1}{2}$ teaspoon soy sauce. Set aside to macerate.

6. Serve the adobo chicken and vegetables with the rice and marinated tomatoes alongside.

TIP

Be sure to tear the soy chicken or seitan into shreds or bite-size chunks so that each forkful is easy to chew.

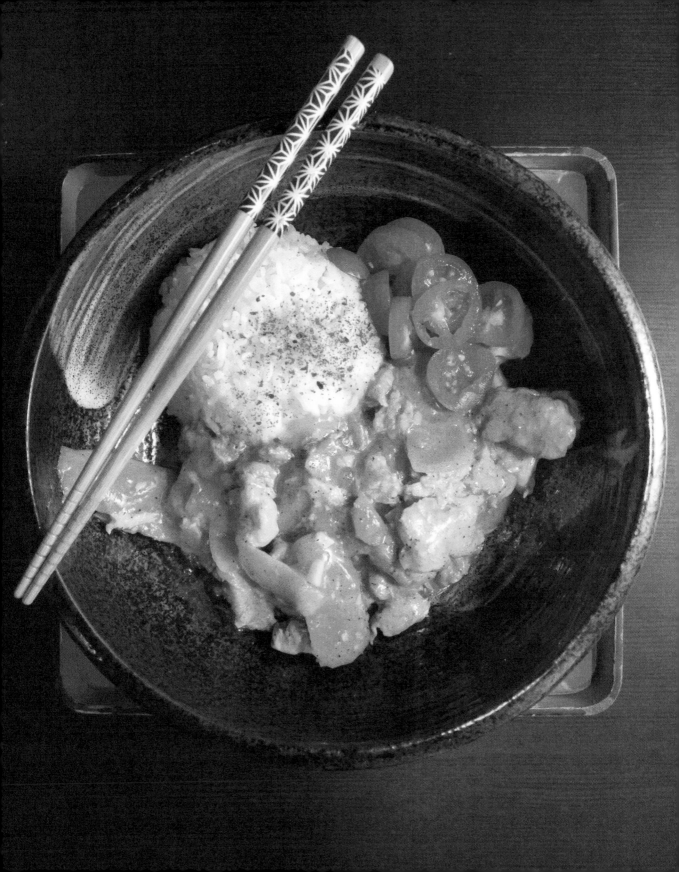

From Donna Jean in San Diego, California

CAST-IRON MAC 'N' CHEESE

SERVES 4 TO 6 • PREP TIME 10 MIN • COOKING TIME 20 TO 25 MIN
TOTAL TIME 30 TO 35 MIN

Ordering vegan mac 'n' cheese at a restaurant is notoriously a gamble. With the plethora of vegan cheese options out there and the infinite possibilities of cashew cheese, soy cheese, coconut cheese, it's impossible to predict if it'll be mouth-watering or mouth-horrifying for my palate. And that's why I wanted to include a recipe for a version I know and love, but also one that . . . wait for it . . . doesn't have any processed cheese in it at all! Wait a second—a hearty, cheesy, satisfying, space-bound-adventure-in-your-mouth mac 'n' cheese without any processed ingredients? How can that be? Read (and cook) the recipe below to find out, and I promise you will not be disappointed. And even harder to believe: Every ingredient in this recipe is actually good for you.

Sea salt

1 pound medium pasta shells

4 tablespoons neutral oil, such as grapeseed or safflower

1 medium yellow onion, chopped

2 ½ cups raw cashew pieces, soaked in water to cover for 1 hour and drained

2 teaspoon smoked paprika

1 teaspoon garlic powder

¼ cup nutritional yeast

2 teaspoon apple cider vinegar

2 plum tomatoes, chopped

1 scallion, thinly sliced, for serving

1. Preheat the oven to 500°F with a rack placed in the center.

2. Bring a large pot of salted water to a boil. Add the pasta and cook until very al dente, 2 to 3 minutes less than directed on the package. Drain the pasta, return it to the pot, and toss with 2 teaspoons of the oil to prevent the pasta from sticking.

3. Meanwhile, in a medium skillet, heat 1 tablespoon of the oil over medium-high heat. Add the onion and cook, stirring, until softened and lightly browned, 3 to 4 minutes. Remove rom the heat and let cool.

4. In a blender, combine the drained cashews, paprika, garlic powder, nutritional yeast, vinegar, the remaining oil, and 4 cups water. Blend until smooth and creamy. Season with salt.

5. Add the cooled onion to the blender and blend until smooth, about 3 minutes.

6. Pour the cashew cheese sauce over the pasta in the pot, and add the tomatoes. Toss until well coated. Transfer the pasta and all the sauce to a 12-inch cast-iron skillet or ovenproof casserole and spread it into an even layer. Bake the mac 'n' cheese until the sauce is set and the top is browned in spots, 15 to 20 minutes. Remove from the oven and let stand for 5 minutes (the sauce will continue to thicken as it rests). Scatter the scallion over the top and serve.

SZECHUAN BEEF

SERVES 6   PREP TIME 30 MIN   COOKING TIME 15 MIN   TOTAL TIME 45 MIN

There aren't many vegan butcher shops around the globe, so I'm proud to say that one of the first in North America exists in my hometown, Toronto. As a plant-based consumer, I do miss that feeling of walking into a butcher shop and having the option of choosing from different varieties of meats, sausages, poultry, and prepared foods. Well, thank God that places like YamChops, where you can purchase prepared plant-based ribs, meatballs, and flavored chicken strips alongside frozen and packaged foods, are starting to become more and more popular. One of their prepared meals that really stuck out to me was their Szechuan beef, which they make in house as a stir-fry over rice. It's filled with sautéed veggies and cooked with a delicious sauce, and the "beef" tastes just like the real thing. All you need to make it at home is your favorite vegan beef or plant-based protein strips.

½ cup soy sauce

½ cup vegetable broth

½ cup cane sugar

¼ cup finely chopped fresh ginger

¼ cup agave syrup

2 tablespoons rice vinegar

1 tablespoon mirin

1 tablespoon sambal oelek

⅓ cup plus 1 ½ teaspoons cornstarch

1 ¼ pounds seitan strips, or 2 ½ (8-ounce) packages other plant-based protein strips, soaked, according to the package directions and patted dry

2 tablespoons grapeseed oil, plus more for frying

1 large yellow onion, halved and thinly sliced lengthwise

1 red bell pepper, cut into thin strips

4 ounces broccoli crowns, cut into ½-inch florets

Steamed brown rice, for serving

1 tablespoon toasted sesame seeds, for garnish

1 scallion, thinly sliced, for garnish

1   In a blender, combine the soy sauce, broth, sugar, ginger, agave syrup, vinegar, mirin, sambal oelek, and 1 ½ teaspoons of the cornstarch. Blend until smooth, then set aside.

2   Put the remaining ⅓ cup cornstarch in a large ziptop bag. Add the seitan strips to the bag, seal it, and shake to coat. Transfer the seitan to a plate, shaking off any excess cornstarch.

3   Fill a large nonstick skillet with ⅛ inch of oil and heat the oil over medium-high heat. Line a plate with a paper towel. Add the seitan strips to the hot oil, in batches so as not to crowd the pan, and cook, turning occasionally, until crispy, about 2 minutes. Transfer to the prepared plate to drain. Add additional oil to the skillet as needed and repeat to cook the remaining seitan strips.

4   Carefully discard the oil, then rinse and dry the skillet. Heat the 2 tablespoons oil over medium-high heat until shimmering. Add the onion, bell pepper, and broccoli and cook, stirring occasionally, until slightly softened and browned in spots, 3 to 4 minutes.

5   Add the cooked seitan strips to the skillet and cook until the vegetables are tender, about 2 minutes more. Add the sauce and cook, stirring, until the sauce thickens and coats the seitan strips and vegetables, 2 to 3 minutes.

6   Serve the seitan and vegetables over brown rice, garnished with the sesame seeds and scallion.

TIP

Instead of brown rice, you can substitute quinoa or your favorite grain!

STRANGER WINGS PIZZA

SERVES 2 TO 4   **PREP TIME 20 MIN**   **COOKING TIME 50 MIN**   **TOTAL TIME 1 HR 10 MIN**

My favorite food on the planet Earth has to be pizza! So you can imagine, when I first went vegan I was like an elephant who no longer lived in a world with peanuts—what was I going to do?! I've searched and searched and am pretty confident I can tell you where to find the best plant-based pizza in any city in North America, and in Vancouver, those pies belong to Virtuous Pie. We're talking Buffalo cauliflower (all the rage right now), bianca sauce, blue cheeze drizzle, all on a perfectly cooked pizza dough! This pizza is tangy from the Buffalo dressing, savory because of the béchamel sauce, and oh-so-hearty with that fried cauliflower. With this particular recipe in my repertoire, I no longer feel like an elephant without peanuts, but like a mammoth—a mammoth who only consumes pizza!

FOR THE BUFFALO CAULIFLOWER

Sunflower oil, for coating

¼ cup all-purpose flour or chickpea flour

1 teaspoon paprika

½ teaspoon onion powder

1 teaspoon garlic powder

½ teaspoon sea salt

½ teaspoon freshly ground black pepper

½ head cauliflower, cut into florets

¼ cup barbecue sauce

¼ cup sriracha

FOR THE "BLUE CHEESE" DRESSING

½ cup vegan mayonnaise

1 tablespoon tahini

1 tablespoon apple cider vinegar

½ teaspoon onion powder

½ teaspoon garlic powder

1 tablespoon nutritional yeast

1 tablespoon freshly squeezed lemon juice

FOR THE BÉCHAMEL SAUCE

1 tablespoon vegan butter

1 tablespoon all-purpose flour

1 cup nondairy milk

Sea salt and freshly ground black pepper

FOR THE PIZZAS

2 tablespoons sunflower oil, plus more for greasing

All-purpose flour, for dusting

1 pound prepared vegan pizza dough, thawed overnight, if frozen, at room temperature

1 shallot, thinly sliced

1 scallion, thinly sliced

1. Preheat the oven to 425°F with rack in upper and lower third of oven. Lightly coat a rimmed baking sheet with oil and place it on the center rack to preheat.

2. In a large bowl, combine the flour, paprika, onion powder, garlic powder, salt, pepper, and ¼ cup water; whisk until smooth. Add the cauliflower and toss to coat.

3. Using oven mitts, remove the preheated baking sheet from the oven and spread the cauliflower over it (the pan should sizzle when the cauliflower makes contact). Bake until the coating forms a crust and the cauliflower is golden underneath, about 20 minutes.

4. Meanwhile, in a large bowl, whisk together the BBQ sauce and sriracha. Add the hot cauliflower and toss to coat, then return the coated cauliflower to the baking sheet and spread it into an even layer. Bake until the sauce is sticky and clings to the cauliflower, 15 to 20 minutes. Remove the cauliflower from the oven and set aside; increase the oven temperature to 450°F.

5. Meanwhile, make the "blue cheese" dressing: In a blender, combine the mayo, tahini, vinegar, onion powder, garlic powder, nutritional yeast, and lemon juice. Blend until smooth; set aside.

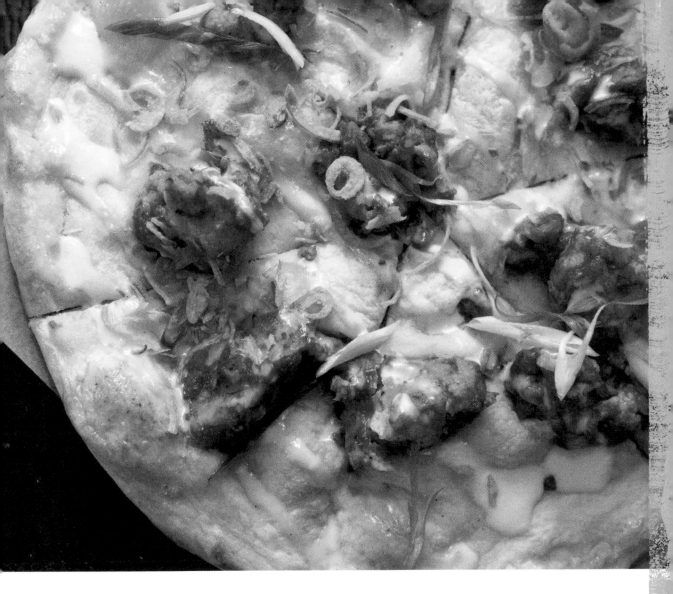

6   Make the béchamel sauce: In a small skillet, melt the butter over medium-high heat. Whisk in the flour until smooth. Slowly whisk in the milk and cook, whisking continuously, until thickened enough to cling to the back of a spoon, about 2 minutes. Season with salt and pepper.

7   Make the pizzas: Lightly grease two 12-inch round pizza pans with oil. Divide the pizza dough in half. On a lightly floured surface, roll each piece into a 12-inch round. Transfer to the prepared pans. Spread the béchamel sauce over each round of dough, leaving a 1-inch border. Bake on the upper and lower oven racks, switching pans halfway through, until the crust is golden and the sauce is golden and bubbling, 8 to 10 minutes.

8   Meanwhile, in a medium skillet, heat the oil over medium-high heat. Add the shallot and cook until golden and crisp. Transfer to a paper towel–lined plate to drain.

9   Top the pizza crusts evenly with the Buffalo cauliflower and the fried shallot. Drizzle with the "blue cheese" dressing, garnish with the scallion, and serve.

CRISPY TOFU TACO & SWEET POTATO TACO

SERVES **4**   PREP TIME **30 TO 40 MIN**   COOKING TIME **15 TO 20 MIN**
TOTAL TIME **45 TO 60 MINUTES**

There ain't no party like a taco party! In my household, tacos are on the menu almost every week. Not only are they nutritious, but the possibilities are endless. Which is why, when we walked into the hole-in-the-wall atmosphere of Taco Party, I didn't really know what to expect. Sure, you can buy some alternative meat and make a pretty mean taco, but what impressed me the most about this place was that all their offerings use whole ingredients. I kid you not, this tofu taco is one of the best I've ever had, vegan or not! The mango salsa, cashew crema, and crispy tofu were a combination only a taco expert could come up with, and the sweet potato tacos were also a home run. So. Have you made plans for next Tuesday yet?

FOR THE SLAW
1 small red cabbage, cored and shredded

¼ cup rice wine vinegar

1 teaspoon cane sugar

Pinch of sea salt

FOR THE MANGO SALSA
1 ripe mango, pitted, peeled, and diced

1 small red onion, finely chopped

1 jalapeño, seeded and diced

1 garlic clove, finely chopped

1 tablespoon freshly squeezed lime juice

2 teaspoons finely chopped fresh cilantro

Sea salt and freshly ground black pepper

FOR THE TOFU TACO FILLING
2 cups vegan panko bread crumbs

2 teaspoons smoked paprika

½ teaspoon garlic powder

Sea salt and freshly ground black pepper

1 cup all-purpose flour

8 ounces extra-firm tofu, drained, patted dry, and cut into ½-inch-thick strips

FOR THE SWEET POTATO TACO FILLING
1 cup rice flour

½ teaspoon ground cinnamon

Sea salt and freshly ground black pepper

1 sweet potato, peeled, halved lengthwise, and thinly sliced into half-moons

TO ASSEMBLE AND SERVE
Neutral oil, for frying

Cashew Crema (page 41)

Corn tortillas, warmed

1 romaine heart, thinly sliced

3 scallions, thinly sliced

1. Make the slaw: In a large bowl, toss together the cabbage, vinegar, sugar, and salt. Set aside to macerate.

2. Make the mango salsa: In a food processor, combine the mango, onion, jalapeño, garlic, and lime juice. Pulse a few times until finely chopped but not pureed. Transfer the salsa to a bowl, stir in the cilantro, season with salt and pepper, and set aside.

3. Make the tofu taco filling: In a shallow bowl, combine the panko, paprika, and garlic powder; season with salt and pepper. In a separate shallow bowl, whisk together the flour and ½ cup water to form a thick batter. Dip the tofu strips into the batter, letting any excess drip off, then press it into the panko, flipping to coat both sides completely.

4. Make the sweet potato taco filling: Combine the rice flour and cinnamon in a ziptop bag; season with salt and pepper. Add the sweet potato slices, seal the bag, and toss to coat. Transfer the sweet potatoes to a baking sheet, shaking off excess flour.

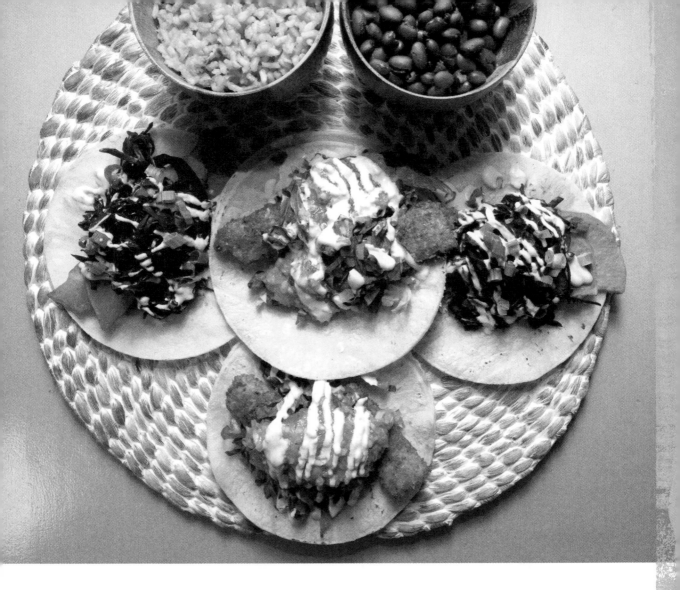

5 Fill a large skillet with ¼ inch of oil and heat the oil over medium-high heat. Line two plates with paper towels. Add the tofu to the hot oil and cook, turning occasionally, until deeply golden all over, 3 to 4 minutes. Transfer to one of the prepared plates to drain.

6 Add more oil to the pan, if needed. When the oil is hot, working in batches, add the sweet potato slices and cook, flipping once, until golden on both sides, 2 to 3 minutes per side. Transfer to the second prepared plate to drain.

7 Set out the tofu, sweet potatoes, cashew crema, tortillas, lettuce, and scallions family-style to assemble as you like!

Make big batches of the cabbage slaw, mango salsa, and cashew crema, and experiment with different tacos at home!

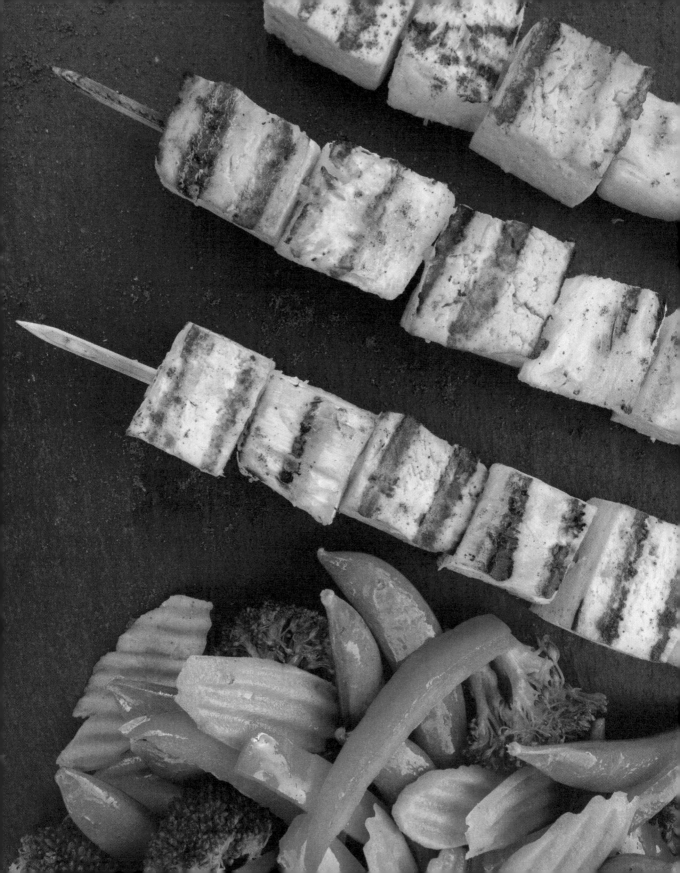

TOFU SKEWERS

SERVES 4   PREP TIME 20 MIN, PLUS 30 MIN MARINATING
COOKING TIME 8 TO 15 MIN   TOTAL TIME 58 TO 65 MIN

A lot of my friends are freaked out by soy and what it does to our bodies. I am here to tell you that unless you're clinically allergic to soy, it's all marketing! Remember when eggs weren't good for us, and then all of a sudden, they had the "good" kind of cholesterol? Or when one cup of milk a day was a necessity to "build healthy bones"? It's MARKETING. Now, I'm not a doctor, but from what I've researched, in my personal opinion, unless you're consuming more than three servings of soy a day, you need not worry. And these tofu skewers are too tasty to fear. I often like to treat tofu like chicken, and this recipe is a perfect example. I highly recommend you make these the day before and let them sit in the fridge to soak up all those juices and flavors, the same way you would marinate chicken overnight. The next day, throw them on the grill with your veggies and you have a delicious, low-calorie, BBQ'd meal. And let's be honest, BBQ'd anything is good for you, duh!

---

2 tablespoons tamari

2 tablespoons pineapple juice

1 teaspoon apple cider vinegar

2 teaspoons finely grated fresh ginger

2 garlic cloves, finely chopped

1/2 teaspoon ground turmeric

1 (14-ounce) package extra-firm tofu, drained, patted dry, and cut into 1 1/2-inch cubes

1 medium carrot, sliced

1 red bell pepper, sliced

4 ounces broccoli crowns, cut into florets

2 ounces snow peas (about 1 cup), ends trimmed

1 tablespoon avocado oil, plus more for greasing

Sea salt and freshly ground black pepper

2 cups cubed fresh pineapple

Handful of fresh cilantro leaves, for garnish

2 scallions, thinly sliced, for garnish

1   In a large bowl, whisk together the tamari, pineapple juice, vinegar, ginger, garlic, and turmeric to combine well.

2   Add the tofu to the marinade and toss to coat. Cover the bowl with plastic wrap and marinate in the refrigerator for at least 30 minutes or up to 24 hours.

3   About 20 minutes before serving, preheat the broiler with a rack positioned 6 inches from the heat source.

4   In a large bowl, toss together the carrot, bell pepper, broccoli, snow peas, and oil. Season with salt and pepper. Spread the vegetables into a single layer on a rimmed baking sheet. Broil the vegetables, stirring occasionally, until tender and browned in spots, 5 to 10 minutes (broiler strengths vary, so watch closely to make sure the vegetables don't burn). Remove the pan from the broiler and cover loosely with aluminum foil to keep warm; keep the broiler on.

5   Lightly grease a second rimmed baking sheet with oil. Remove the tofu from the marinade. Skewer alternating pieces of tofu and pineapple on 4 skewers, placing them on the prepared baking sheet as you go. Broil, turning the skewers occasionally, until the tofu and pineapple are browned in spots, 3 to 5 minutes.

6   Serve the skewers and vegetables garnished with the cilantro and scallions.

TIPS

Make sure you completely drain and dry your tofu, or it won't absorb the marinade as well.

If using wooden skewers, soak them for 20 minutes first to prevent burning. Instead of broiling the vegetables and skewers, you can put the vegetables on a sheet of aluminum foil, wrap it around them to make a packet, and cook them alongside the assembled skewers on an outdoor grill.

ETHIOPIAN DINNER

SERVES 4   PREP TIME 45 MIN   COOK TIME 1 HR   TOTAL TIME 1 HR 45 MIN

As close as Ethiopia is to Egypt, it's surprising that I haven't experienced much Ethiopian cuisine at all. But what better place to try some vegan Ethiopian food than New York City? Bunna Cafe, an all-Ethiopian spot located in Brooklyn, is serving up all of the country's staples, from coffee to *t'ej*, an authentic golden honey wine, to *misir wat*, the red lentil mash you see here. Bunna has graciously provided recipes from their kitchen that have been passed down from generation to generation. What I learned from my short time at Bunna is that many of their recipes start with their ginger-garlic paste, the recipe for which you can find on the following page (and which you can prepare up to a week in advance). This paste is combined with split peas, lentils, or even collard greens and cabbage. This base allows for a flavoring that is authentic to Ethiopian cuisine. So no matter what you decide to serve up for this Ethiopian fest, make sure you have plenty of ginger and garlic to go around!

FOR THE YELLOW SPLIT PEAS

2 tablespoons safflower oil

1 small red onion, chopped

1/2 teaspoon sea salt

1 teaspoon ground turmeric

1 very ripe plum tomato, chopped

1 tablespoon Ginger-Garlic Paste (recipe follows)

1 cup dried yellow split peas, rinsed and drained

FOR THE MISIR WAT

3 tablespoons safflower oil

1 medium red onion, chopped

1/2 teaspoon sea salt

2 tablespoons berbere spice blend

1 very ripe plum tomato, chopped

1 tablespoon Ginger-Garlic Paste (recipe follows)

2/3 cup dried red lentils, rinsed and drained

FOR THE ATKILT WAT

3 tablespoons safflower oil

1 small green cabbage, cored and shredded

2 medium carrots, shredded

2 Yukon Gold potatoes, peeled and cut into chunks

1/2 teaspoon sea salt

1/2 teaspoon ground turmeric

1 tablespoon Ginger-Garlic Paste (recipe follows)

FOR THE COLLARD GREENS

3 tablespoons safflower oil

2 tablespoons Ginger-Garlic Paste (recipe follows)

1 bunch collard greens, stemmed, leaves chopped into thin strips

1/2 teaspoon sea salt

Pinch of ground cardamom

Injera bread, for serving

1   Make the yellow split peas: In a medium pot, heat the oil over medium heat. Add the onion and salt and cook, stirring, until softened, 2 to 3 minutes. Add the turmeric, tomato, and ginger-garlic paste and cook until fragrant, 1 to 2 minutes. Add the split peas and 2 cups water. Bring to a boil, then reduce the heat to medium-low and simmer until the peas are tender but still intact, adding more water as needed to prevent them from drying out, about 20 minutes.

2   At the same time, get the misir wat going: In a separate medium pot, heat the oil over medium heat. Add the onion and salt and cook, stirring, until softened, 2 to 3 minutes. Add the berbere, tomato, and ginger-garlic paste and cook until fragrant, 1 to 2 minutes. Add the lentils and 2 cups water. Bring to a boil, then reduce the heat to medium-low and simmer until the lentils are tender but still intact, adding more water as needed to prevent them from drying out, about 20 minutes.

3   Meanwhile, make the atkilt wat: In a large skillet, heat the oil over medium-high heat. Add the cabbage, carrots, potatoes, and salt. Cover and cook until the cabbage begins to wilt, about 2 minutes. Stir in the turmeric and ginger-garlic paste. Reduce the heat to medium and cook, stirring occasionally, until the cabbage reduces in volume and both the cabbage and potatoes are tender, about 10 minutes. Remove from the heat and let cool.

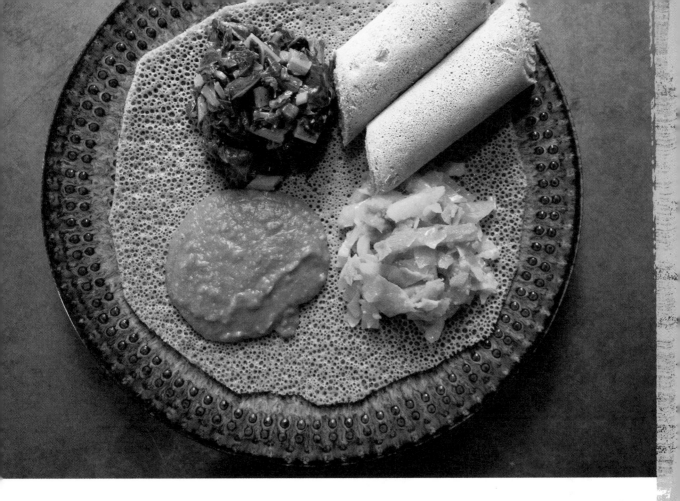

4. Make the collard greens: In a large skillet, heat the oil over medium-high heat until shimmering. Add the ginger-garlic paste and cook until fragrant, about 1 minute. Add the collard greens, salt, and cardamom. Cook, stirring, until wilted and just tender (they will be much more toothsome than American-style collard greens), about 5 minutes.

5. Arrange the yellow split peas, misir wat, atkilt wat, and collard greens in separate serving bowls and serve family-style, with injera alongside.

TIP

You can buy injera online, but store-bought buckwheat crepes or roti, while different, can be substituted.

GINGER-GARLIC PASTE

2 heads garlic, cloves
separated and peeled

2 (4-inch) pieces fresh ginger,
peeled and finely grated

½ cup safflower oil

Combine the garlic cloves, ginger, and oil in a food processor or blender and process into a paste. Store in an airtight container in the refrigerator for up to 1 week.

INDIAN TOFU CURRY

SERVES 2 TO 4   **PREP TIME** 15 MIN   **COOKING TIME** 22 TO 25 MIN   **TOTAL TIME** 37 TO 40 MIN

I have a special place in my heart for Indian food, as I'm sure most of you do. Not only is it innately plant-based, but the use of spices and aromas is unparalleled. Indian food has become a big part of my rotation in the kitchen lately because I get to learn about and cook with all of these aromatic spices. It makes my kitchen smell delicious! Curries from Southeast Asia are incredibly popular in North America, but to find a basic, flavorful Indian curry can sometimes be difficult, which is why I wanted to include one in this book. The secret is the sunflower seed *saag*, which acts as the base in this curry. Keep in mind that you can replace the tofu in this dish with an array of vegetables or something like chickpeas, and it will turn out just as tasty. So no matter what protein or vegetables you're in the mood for, this dish will have your neighbors sitting outside your door just for the smell!

FOR THE SUNFLOWER SEED SAAG

⅓ cup sunflower seeds

½ jalapeño, seeded (if you prefer less heat) and finely chopped

2 tablespoons coconut oil

1 small yellow onion, sliced

1 garlic clove, finely chopped

1 tablespoon finely chopped fresh ginger

1 teaspoon garam masala

2 teaspoons coriander seeds, toasted

2 teaspoons cumin seeds, toasted

1 teaspoon ground turmeric

Sea salt and freshly ground black pepper

FOR THE CURRY

2 tablespoons coconut oil

1 small red onion, finely chopped

7 ounces extra-firm tofu, drained and cubed

2 cups packed baby spinach

Small handful of fresh cilantro leaves, for garnish

1. Make the sunflower seed saag: Combine the sunflower seeds and 1 ½ cups water in a small saucepan. Bring to a boil over high heat, add the jalapeño, then reduce the heat to medium and simmer until the jalapeño and sunflower seeds are tender, about 10 minutes. Transfer to a blender and let cool.

2. In a medium skillet, melt the coconut oil over medium-high heat. Add the onion and cook until lightly browned, 3 to 4 minutes. Remove from the heat and stir in the garlic and ginger, then spoon the mixture into the blender with the sunflower seeds and jalapeño. Add the garam masala, coriander, cumin, and turmeric to the blender. Blend until smooth. Season with salt and pepper and set aside.

3. Make the curry: In a medium skillet, melt the coconut oil over medium heat. Add the onion and cook until softened, about 3 minutes. Using a slotted spoon, transfer the onion to a plate and set aside.

4. Add the tofu to the empty skillet and cook, turning occasionally, until lightly browned all over, 5 to 6 minutes.

5. Stir in the spinach and cook until slightly wilted, then stir in the sunflower seed saag. Reduce the heat to medium-low and cook until the saag is just heated through, 1 to 2 minutes.

6. Spoon the curry into individual bowls and garnish with cilantro. Serve immediately.

SPANISH RICE & SAUSAGE FAJITA

SERVES 4 TO 6   PREP TIME 15 MIN   COOKING TIME 20 TO 25 MIN   TOTAL TIME 35 TO 40 MIN

A while back, I kept hearing about these vegan sausages that everyone was going crazy for, but I had a really hard time finding them. When I finally tracked them down and tried them, I came up with this recipe. Sometimes a single ingredient can inspire you to try something new, and that's exactly what happened with this Spanish rice and sausage fajita. I recommend a hot Italian vegan sausage to go with the slightly sweeter Spanish rice. The sweetness comes from the chipotle in adobo sauce, which contains a little bit of sugar, but the combination of spicy and sweet is fantastic. For even more spice, I add a jalapeño or serrano pepper to the Spanish rice itself, but if you like things on the milder side, feel free to skip it. But just know that if you do, you're a wuss. Just kidding. But really, leave it in.

FOR THE SPANISH RICE

2 tablespoons avocado oil

1 white onion, diced

4 garlic cloves, minced

1 jalapeño, diced

2 cups uncooked brown basmati rice

1 (12-ounce) can fire-roasted diced tomatoes

2 tablespoons minced chipotle chiles in adobo sauce

2 tablespoons tomato paste

2 cups vegetable broth

1 teaspoon sea salt

FOR THE SAUSAGE FAJITA

1 tablespoon avocado oil

½ red onion, thinly sliced into half-moons

4 garlic cloves, minced

Sea salt and freshly ground black pepper

½ poblano pepper, thinly sliced

½ red bell pepper, thinly sliced

½ yellow bell pepper, thinly sliced

1 jalapeño, thinly sliced (optional)

4 vegan sausage links (I like Buzz Lightyear's Hot Italian—think about it), sliced

Lime wedges, for garnish

Fresh cilantro leaves, for garnish

1. Make the Spanish rice: Preheat the oven to 350°F. In a Dutch oven, heat the avocado oil over medium heat. Add the onion, garlic, and jalapeño and cook for 3 to 5 minutes, until the onion softens. Add the rice and cook until the rice is lightly toasted, about 3 minutes. Add the tomatoes and chipotle chiles and cook for 2 minutes more.

2. Add the tomato paste and broth and stir well to combine. Season with the salt and bring to a boil. Cover the Dutch oven and place in the oven. Bake for 15 minutes, then stir, cover, and cook for 15 minutes more, or until the liquid has been fully absorbed and the rice is cooked.

3. Meanwhile, make the sausage fajita: In a pan, heat the oil over medium-low heat. Add the onion and garlic. Season with salt and black pepper and stir. Add the poblano, bell peppers, and jalapeño, raise the heat to medium, and cook for 3 to 5 minutes.

4. Raise the heat to medium-high, add the sausage, and cook for about 5 minutes, until the veggies and sausage are nicely browned but not burned.

5. Remove the rice from the oven, squeeze a wedge of lime on top of the rice, and add the sausage fajita. Garnish with a few more lime wedges and a sprinkle of cilantro, and serve.

TIP

For extra flavor, serve with guacamole and/or your favorite vegan sour cream.

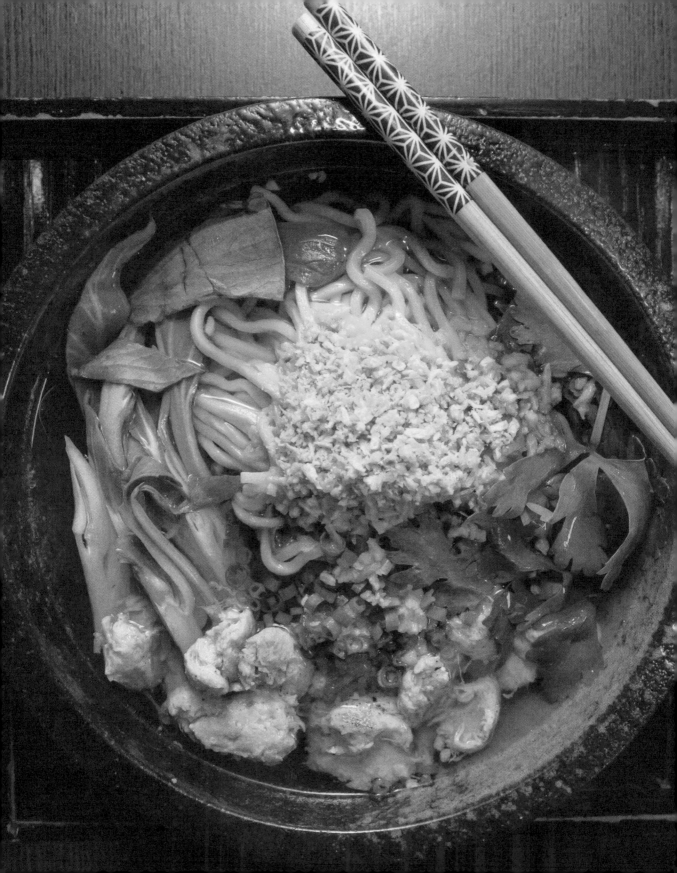

MAMI
NOODLE SOUP

SERVES 2   PREP TIME **15 MIN**   COOK TIME **75 MIN**   TOTAL TIME **90 MIN**

I don't care what the doctor prescribes or what ancient oil your friend says you should use when you're sick or trying to prevent an illness—there is nothing that will make you feel better than a homemade noodle soup. This traditional Taiwanese "chicken" noodle bowl takes that home remedy to another level! It features hearty noodles, tons of bok choy, cilantro, fried scallions, and a broth that will have you feeling like Iron Man 3000. (Thanks, Downey.) When I first tried this dish at Ichiza it blew my mind, and no, it wasn't the habanero chile oil that I added to it—it was just that good! So unless you're in Portland and can try this dish from the owner, Cyrus Ichiza, himself, there is no better noodle soup you can make than this one right here.

4 cups water, plus more as needed

1 pound vegan soy chicken or seitan, shredded or crumbled into large pieces

3 scallions, halved crosswise, plus 1 sliced for garnish

6 slices fresh ginger

4 pods star anise

¼ cup coconut oil

3 cloves garlic

1 red chile, halved lengthwise, plus 1 red chile, finely diced, for garnish

½ medium white onion, sliced

½ tablespoon coconut sugar

1½ tablespoons bean paste

½ cup liquid aminos

1/4 cup rice wine vinegar

4 grape tomatoes, halved

1 teaspoon sea salt

1 teaspoon freshly ground black pepper

1 dried bay leaf

2 bundles rice noodles

2 cups bok choy

½ cup fresh cilantro

1 tablespoon fried onion, for garnish

1. Put 4 cups of water, the soy chicken, 6 scallion halves, 3 slices of ginger, and 2 star anise pods into a medium pot. Bring to a boil and cook for 5 minutes. Remove from the heat.

2. Meanwhile, add the coconut oil to a large wok with the remaining sliced scallion, ginger, and star anise pods, as well as the garlic, red chile, and onion. Stir for 1 minute. Add the coconut sugar and stir for 30 seconds.

3. Using a slotted spoon, remove the soy chicken and set aside. Reserve the pot with the water and vegetables.

4. Add the bean paste to the wok and stir well. Add the soy chicken, the liquid aminos, and vinegar, and stir. Add the tomatoes and cook for 10 minutes, stirring every minute or so.

5. Transfer the mixture in the wok to the reserved pot. Add the salt, pepper, and bay leaf to the pot and cover. Place over low heat and simmer for 60 minutes.

6. Meanwhile, prepare the rice noodles: Bring a pot of water to a boil. Add the rice noodles and cook according to the package instructions, likely 5 to 7 minutes. Transfer the noodles to a strainer with tongs, and keep the water in the pot.

7. Bring the water back to a boil and add the bok choy. Blanch for 1 minute, then remove with the ladle.

8. Divide the noodles, bok choy, and soy chicken between two serving bowls. Using a soup ladle, add broth to each bowl, according to your preference.

9. Top with the sliced scallions, diced red chile, cilantro, and fried onions and serve.

TIPS

If you do not have a wok, use a deep pan or pot.

For more spice, add another red chile or two.

KOSHARE

SERVES 4 TO 6   **PREP TIME 20 MIN, PLUS OVERNIGHT SOAKING**
COOKING TIME 30 MIN   **TOTAL TIME 50 MIN**

This has to be one of my favorite meals of all time. But I warn you, this is not a dish you want to be eating if you're watching your calories. We're talking two different kinds of pasta on top of a rice-lentil mix, topped with chickpeas and drenched in a rich tomato sauce. But I promise you it's worth it. Growing up, before I was actually plant-based, this was my favorite (unknowingly) vegan meal. My sisters and I would request this dish from my mom on a regular basis. In Egypt, it's one of the most common street foods, and a lot of vendors serve it up in a plastic sandwich bag, tie it tight, and rip the corner off so it acts like a piping funnel. That's how good this dish is—what other food could possibly drive a nation of 100 million people to literally funnel it into their mouths with a homemade piping bag? No other food. None. That's the answer.

FOR THE LENTILS, RICE, AND PASTA

2 teaspoons sea salt, plus more as needed

¼ cup plus 1 tablespoon safflower or sunflower oil

2 large yellow onions, halved and thinly sliced through the root end

1 cup dried brown lentils, rinsed, soaked in water for at least 3 hours or up to overnight, then drained

2 ½ cups jasmine rice, rinsed until the water runs mostly clear

1 tablespoon ground cumin

½ teaspoon chili powder

1 cup uncooked elbow pasta or ditalini

1 cup uncooked broken spaghetti noodles

FOR THE SAUCE

2 tablespoons safflower or sunflower oil

6 garlic cloves, minced

1 tablespoon ground cumin

1 ½ teaspoons paprika

1 ½ tablespoons ground coriander

1 tablespoon chili powder

1 (24-ounce) jar tomato passata or crushed tomatoes

1 tablespoon white wine vinegar

Sea salt and freshly ground black pepper

1 (15-ounce) can chickpeas, drained and rinsed, for serving

1. Make the lentils, rice, and pasta: Bring a large pot of salted water to a boil.

2. Meanwhile, in a large skillet, heat ¼ cup of the oil over medium-high heat. Add the onions and cook, stirring occasionally, until deep golden brown, 8 to 10 minutes. Use a slotted spoon to transfer the onions to a paper towel–lined plate. Carefully discard the oil and set the skillet aside (no need to rinse it).

3. In a large pot, combine the lentils, rice, cumin, salt, chili powder, ¼ cup of the fried onions, (reserve the rest for serving), and 4 cups water. Bring to a boil over high heat, then reduce the heat to low, cover, and cook until the rice and lentils are tender and the water has mostly evaporated.

4. Add both pastas to the boiling water and cook according to the package directions until al dente. Drain the pasta, return it to the pot, and toss with the remaining 1 tablespoon oil (this prevents the pasta from sticking).

5. Meanwhile, make the sauce: In the skillet you used to cook the onions, heat the oil over medium-high heat. Add the garlic and cook until golden and fragrant, about 1 minute.

6. Add the cumin, paprika, coriander, and chili powder, then stir in the tomatoes and vinegar; season with salt and black pepper. Bring to a boil, then reduce the heat to medium. Cook for about 5 minutes, until the sauce has reduced slightly.

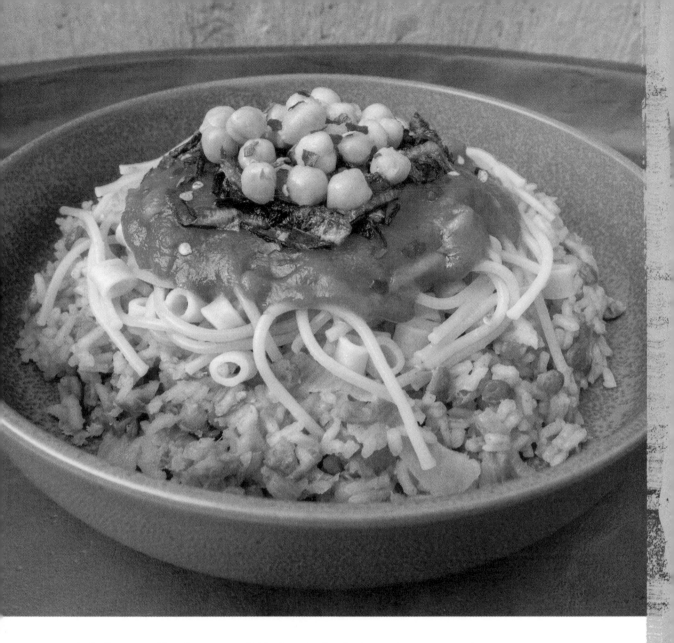

7   Divide the rice and lentils among individual serving bowls. Spoon the pasta over, then top with the sauce. Top with the chickpeas and the remaining fried onions and serve.

TIPS

Soak the lentils the night before to avoid having to wait for them to soak.

If you can't find tomato passata, use regular crushed tomatoes and add 1 to 2 tablespoons tomato paste to thicken it up.

Instead of discarding the oil you used for the onion, you can let it cool and save it in an airtight container for future frying.

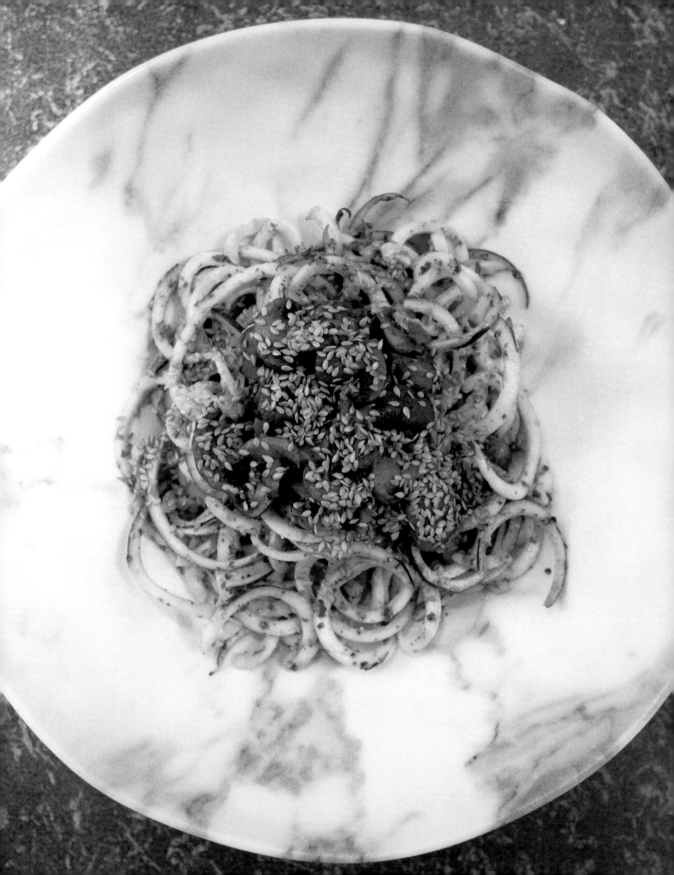

LE MADRID ZUCCHINI NOODLES

SERVES **2**   PREP TIME **15 MIN**   COOKING TIME **10 MIN**   TOTAL TIME **25 MIN**

I love myself a vegetable noodle! Ever since the invention of the spiralizer, vegetable noodles have become an increasingly popular ingredient in the culinary world. The best part about this recipe is the walnut. You can use it on zucchini noodles like this, on a more traditional pasta, or on a selection of vegetables. Try it with spiralized carrots, spaghetti squash, or even sweet potatoes. No matter what vegetable you try, I promise you this will be the best healthy alternative to a traditional pasta that you can find. Because once in a while, we all need to sub out those carbs for veggies.

FOR THE PESTO
2 cups packed fresh basil leaves

½ cup walnuts, toasted

1 tablespoon freshly squeezed lemon juice

3 tablespoons nutritional yeast

½ cup olive oil

Sea salt and freshly ground black pepper

FOR THE SALAD
1 pound white button mushrooms, sliced

2 tablespoons olive oil

1 garlic clove, finely chopped

Sea salt and freshly ground black pepper

1 tablespoon flaxseeds

½ teaspoon harissa spice mix (not harissa paste)

2 large zucchini, spiralized, or 16 to 20 ounces store-bought zoodles

1. Preheat the oven to 400°F.

2. Make the pesto: In a food processor, combine the basil and walnuts; pulse a few times until the mixture is coarsely ground. Add the lemon juice, nutritional yeast, and 3 tablespoons water. Pulse once or twice to combine. With the food processor running, slowly drizzle in the olive oil and process until smooth. Season with salt and pepper.

3. Make the salad: On a rimmed baking sheet, toss the mushroons with the olive oil and garlic. Season with salt and pepper. Spread the mushrooms into a single layer and roast until tender and golden, about 10 minutes.

4. Meanwhile, in a small skillet, combine the flaxseeds and harissa spice. Cook over medium heat, stirring, until fragrant, 1 to 2 minutes.

5. In a large bowl, toss the zucchini noodles with half the pesto. Top with the mushrooms, sprinkle with the flaxseeds, and serve.

TIP
The pesto will keep well in an airtight container in the fridge for a few days. Top the pesto with a layer of olive oil to prevent browning, if you are not using it the same day.

MARGHERITA PIZZA

MAKES ONE 14-INCH PIZZA **PREP TIME 15 MIN, PLUS 1 TO 1 HR 30 MIN RISING TIME**
COOKING TIM 8 TO 10 MIN **TOTAL TIME 23 TO 25 MIN**

One of the foods I've been most intrigued by in the past year of my plant-based journey is bread dough. Our ancestors, no matter which part of the world you came from, most likely ate bread as a source of sustenance. Now with gluten-intolerance and celiac disease, it's hard to imagine that we used to survive off bread, but research shows that it's the way the ingredients are processed that has led to this outbreak. If you suffer from celiac disease or gluten-intolerance, then please don't try this recipe, but if staying away from gluten is a *preference* and you're craving some pizza, you may want to try this one, which uses high-quality flours. The tipo "00" flour is an Italian-style flour that is commonly used for pizzas in Italy because it has a slightly lower protein content, which results in a smoother dough and more flavorful pizza crust. It's especially perfect for a Margherita pizza because all you have is the dough and the sauce. Like many recipes in this book, this is only a launching pad. Once you feel comfortable making the dough, feel free to play around with the toppings, and even the sauce!

1 teaspoon active dry yeast

½ teaspoon cane sugar

¾ cup warm water (110°F)

2 teaspoons plus 1 tablespoon olive oil, plus more for greasing

2 cups bread flour, plus more for dusting

½ teaspoon sea salt, plus more as needed

1 (14-ounce) can whole peeled tomatoes

1 garlic clove, finely chopped

Freshly ground black pepper

4 ounces vegan mozzarella cheese, cut into cubes

¼ cup shredded vegan parmesan cheese

A few fresh basil leaves, torn

TIP

Antimo Caputo tipo "00" flour is a great upgrade here if you can find it, as it makes for a lighter crust.

1 In a medium bowl, stir together the yeast, sugar, and warm water. Let stand for 5 to 10 minutes, until bubbles start to appear on the surface (this indicates the yeast is active).

2 Add 2 teaspoons of the olive oil, the flour, and salt to the yeast mixture and stir with a wooden spoon until the flour is fully absorbed. Lightly flour the counter or a large cutting board. Scrape the dough onto the floured surface, sprinkle a little more flour over the dough, and knead until smooth, 5 to 7 minutes. Lightly brush the bowl you used for the dough with oil. Put the dough back in the bowl, cover tightly with plastic wrap, and let rest in a warm spot until doubled in volume, 1 to 1 ½ hours.

3 Meanwhile, put the tomatoes in a food processor and process until smooth (or leave them a little chunky, if you prefer).

4 In a small saucepan, heat the remaining 1 tablespoon oil over medium-high heat. Add the garlic and cook until fragrant, about 30 seconds. Add the pureed tomatoes and season with salt and pepper. Reduce the heat to medium-low and simmer until the sauce thickens and reduces slightly, about 5 minutes. Set aside to cool.

5 When the dough is ready, preheat the oven to 500°F with a rack set in the lowest position. Lightly brush a 16-inch round pizza pan with oil.

6 On a lightly floured counter, gently stretch the dough into a 14-inch round (if you feel more comfortable using a rolling pin, then go ahead and use it!). Transfer the dough to the prepared pizza pan.

7 Spread the sauce over the dough, leaving a 1-inch border. Scatter the mozzarella and half the parmesan evenly over the sauce. Bake on the bottom rack until the crust is crisp and golden, and the cheese has melted, 8 to 10 minutes. Top with the remaining parmesan and the basil and serve.

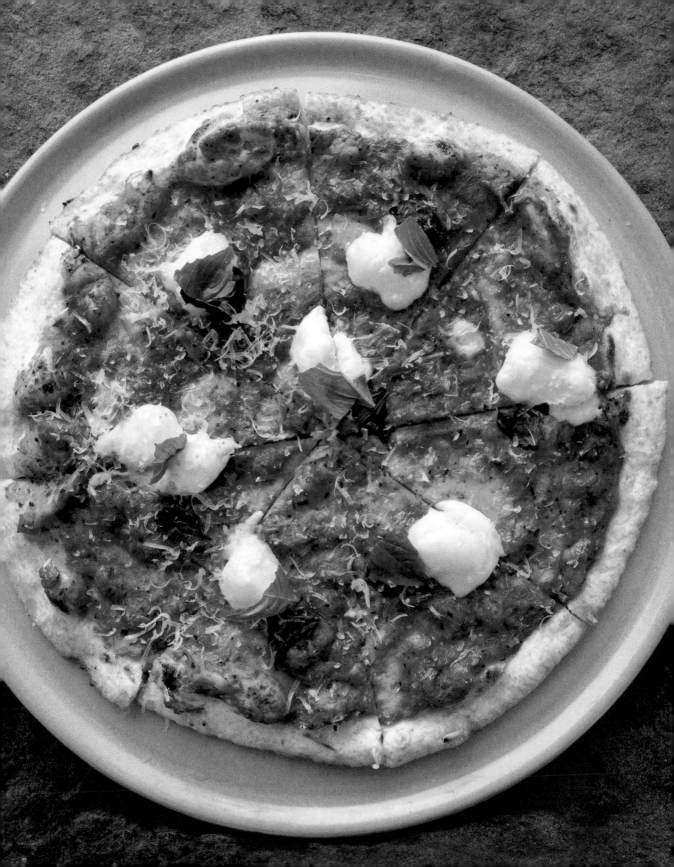

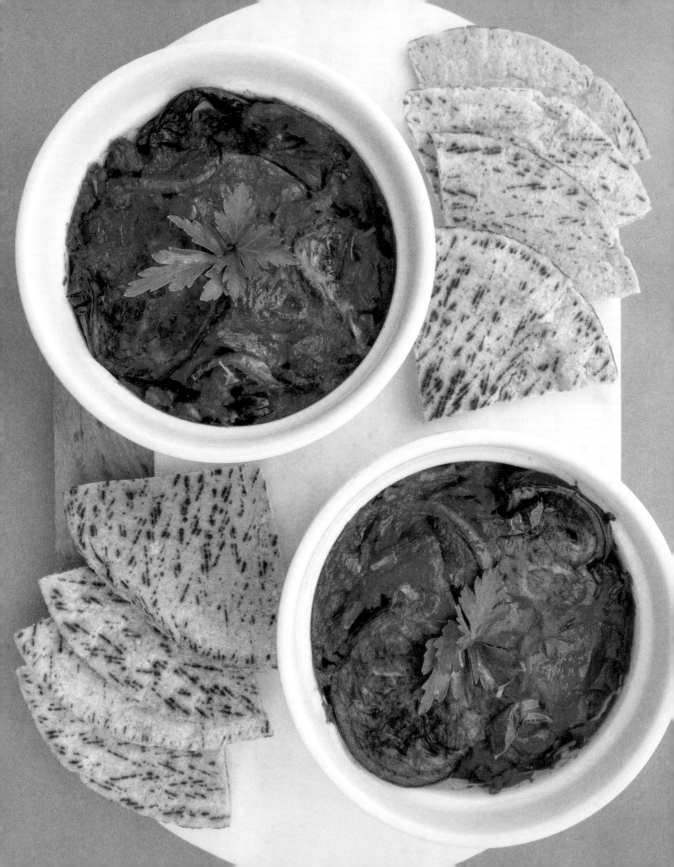

MOUSSAKA (EGGPLANT STEW)

SERVES **4 TO 6**   PREP TIME **10 MIN**   COOKING TIME **40 TO 45 MIN**   TOTAL TIME **ABOUT 1 HR**

Much like *bamya*, the okra stew my mom makes (see page 120), this is a classic Egyptian stew. The real difference between the two recipes is the vegetable being featured. Both take their particular vegetables and transform them into warm and comforting versions of themselves. Another difference is that I prefer this dish with pita bread instead of rice. So in this recipe we've included both options, rice and pita bread, and you can serve both if you like. You also get bell pepper and jalapeño for a little bit of a kick.

- 2 Italian eggplant (about 1 pound total), sliced into ¼-inch-thick rounds
- 2 green bell peppers, cut into strips
- 4 tablespoons olive oil
- Sea salt
- 1 large yellow onion, coarsely chopped
- 3 garlic cloves, chopped
- 1 jalapeño, seeded (if desired) and finely chopped
- 1 tablespoon ground cumin
- 1 tablespoon ground coriander
- 1 (6-ounce) can tomato paste
- Freshly ground black pepper
- Steamed brown basmati rice, for serving
- Warm pita bread, for serving

1. Preheat the oven to 400°F.

2. Put the eggplant and bell peppers on a rimmed baking sheet and toss with 3 tablespoons of the olive oil; season with salt. Spread the vegetables over the baking sheet in a single layer. Bake until tender, 20 to 25 minutes. Remove from the oven; keep the oven on.

3. In a large skillet, heat the remaining 1 tablespoon oil over medium heat. Add the onion, garlic, and jalapeño and cook until fragrant and the onion is slightly softened, 2 to 3 minutes. Stir in the cumin, coriander, tomato paste, and 1 cup water and bring to a boil. Add the eggplant and bell peppers, season with pepper, and stir to coat.

4. Spoon the vegetables and sauce into an 8-inch square baking dish. Bake until slightly thickened and the top is lightly browned, 15 to 20 minutes.

5. Serve hot, with basmati rice and pita bread.

TIP

The best garnish for this dish is some really fine olive oil. Drizzle it on top of the moussaka while it's warm in the baking dish before serving.

BAMYA (OKRA STEW)

SERVES **2 TO 4**   PREP TIME **15 MIN**   COOKING TIME **45 MIN**   TOTAL TIME **1 HR**

My mom was exactly how you would imagine an immigrant mom in the kitchen: a fantastic cook who never really moved away from her culinary roots. She cooked classic Egyptian dinners every night from the minute I was born to the day I moved away from home. She had enough of a culinary arsenal that my sisters and I never got bored of her food, and after I moved out of the house, I began to associate her food with a sense of home. Home isn't so much a physical place, or a city, it's a feeling. Feelings of comfort and warmth, security and familiarity—feelings that I associate with my mother's cooking. On a cold winter day in Toronto, when it's snowing so hard and it's so cold outside that I'm convinced it has to be better living in the Arctic, all I want is to be wrapped in a blanket, eating a bowl of this warm, comforting, tomatoey okra stew and watching a Raptors game. Serve it over some rice or with warm pita bread for dipping.

FOR THE BAMYA

2 tablespoons neutral oil, such as grapeseed or safflower

1 medium yellow onion, diced

5 garlic cloves, diced

1 jalapeño, diced

1 (6-ounce) can tomato paste

1 tablespoon freshly squeezed lemon juice

1 teaspoon ground coriander

Sea salt and freshly ground black pepper

1 pound okra, trimmed (preferably fresh, but frozen is okay, too)

FOR THE EGYPTIAN RICE

2 tablespoons coconut oil

1 cup broken vermicelli noodles

1 1/2 cups white parboiled long-grain rice, rinsed

1 teaspoon sea salt

1   Make the bamya: In a medium pot, heat the oil over medium-high heat. Add the onion, garlic, and jalapeño. Cook, stirring, until the onion is softened and golden, 3 to 5 minutes.

2   Stir in the tomato paste, lemon juice, coriander, and 1/2 cup water. Season with salt and pepper. Increase the heat to high and bring the mixture to a boil. Add the okra, stir to combine, then reduce the heat to low. Cover loosely with a lid (you want to allow some steam to escape) and simmer until the okra is very tender, about 45 minutes.

3   Meanwhile, make the Egyptian rice: In a large saucepan, melt the coconut oil over medium-high heat. Add the vermicelli and cook, stirring continuously, until golden and fragrant, about 3 minutes. Add the rice, salt, and 2 1/4 cups water. Bring to a boil, then cover, reduce the heat to low, and simmer until the water has been mostly absorbed and the rice and vermicelli are tender, about 20 minutes.

4   Taste the okra and season with more salt and pepper, if needed. Serve with the Egyptian rice.

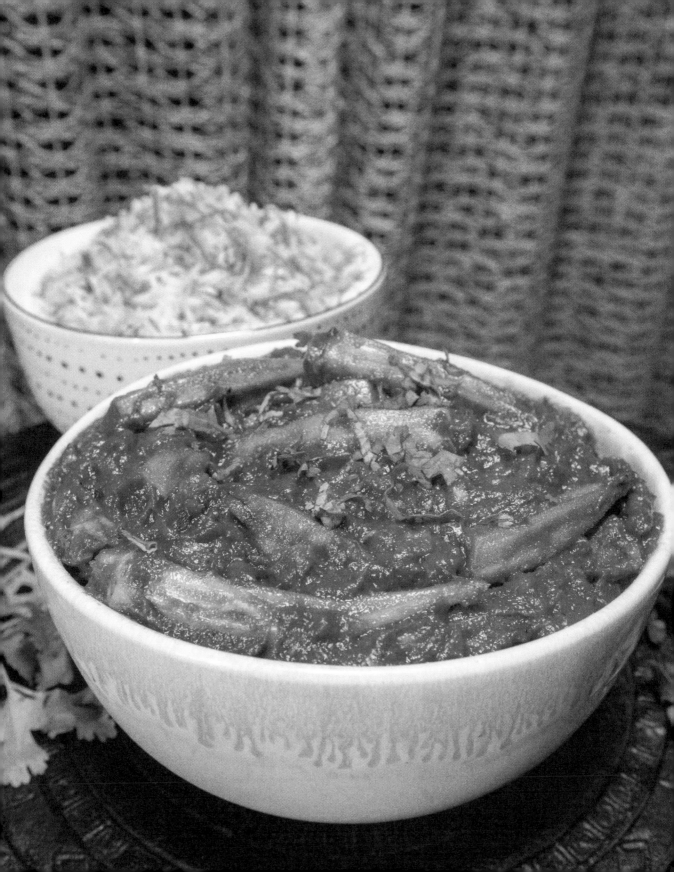

MUSHROOM COUSCOUS

SERVES 2 TO 4   **PREP TIME 15 TO 20 MIN**   **COOKING TIME 15 MIN**   **TOTAL TIME 30 TO 35 MIN**

This dish, another one of my favorites from Aviv, inspired one of Evolving Vegan's bestselling clothing items at: a cropped T-shirt with the saying "cous cous gets me loose loose." Needless to say, we were all in a pretty fun, happy mood during this leg of the tour, and after we visited Aviv and ate their mushroom couscous, we came up with this slogan. And trust me, you'll understand when you try this dish. When cooked correctly, oyster mushrooms have an incredibly meaty texture, and combined with some beautiful couscous, a creamy homemade cashew labneh, and a spicy *harif* (a Middle Eastern chile paste), this dish will satisfy all your cravings. It's a healthy-carb dish with a meaty vegetable, creamy dollops of sauce, and a homemade spice—what more could you possibly need in life? And if you didn't know, couscous is actually a North African "pasta" of sorts, made from wheat!

3/4 teaspoon sea salt

2 cups uncooked pearl couscous

2 teaspoons pomegranate molasses

1 teaspoon white wine vinegar

1/4 teaspoon dried oregano

Pinch of ground nutmeg

2 tablespoons vegan butter

1 medium carrot, thinly sliced

8 ounces oyster mushrooms, any large pieces halved

1/4 bunch Swiss chard, leaves and stems cut into 1-inch pieces

1 1/2 teaspoons Harif (recipe follows)

1/4 cup Cashew Labneh (see page 147)

1/2 teaspoon za'atar, for sprinkling

Edible flowers, for garnish (optional)

1. In a medium saucepan, combine 3 cups water and the salt and bring to a boil over high heat. Add the couscous, reduce the heat to medium-low, cover, and cook until tender and the water has been mostly absorbed, about 15 minutes; drain off any excess water. Cover to keep warm and set aside.

2. Meanwhile, in a small bowl, whisk together the pomegranate molasses, vinegar, oregano, and nutmeg; set aside.

3. In a large skillet, melt 1 tablespoon of the vegan butter over medium-high heat. Add the carrot and cook, stirring, until lightly golden, about 2 minutes. Add 2 tablespoons water, cover, and cook until tender, 2 to 3 minutes. Transfer to a plate.

4. In the same skillet, melt the remaining 1 tablespoon butter over medium-high heat. Add the mushrooms and cook until they are golden and have released some of their liquid. Add the Swiss chard and cook until the leaves are wilted and the stems are barely tender, about 2 minutes.

5. Add the couscous, carrot, harif, and pomegranate molasses mixture. Stir to combine and cook until the couscous is heated through, 1 to 2 minutes more.

6. Spoon the couscous onto plates. Add a dollop of cashew labneh and sprinkle with za'atar. Garnish with edible flowers, if desired, and serve.

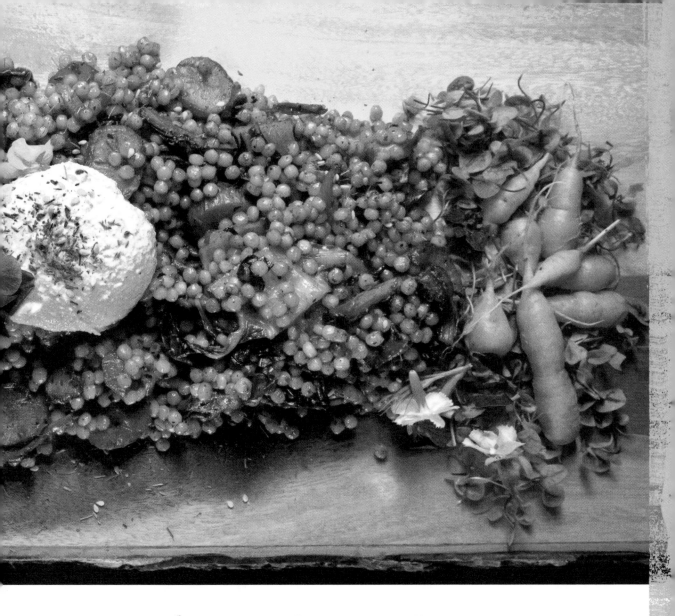

HARIF (MIDDLE EASTERN CHILE PASTE)

2 medium garlic cloves

1 jalapeño

1 1/2 cups rice bran oil
  or other neutral oil

1 cup Aleppo pepper

1 tablespoon Urfa biber
  (Turkish red pepper)
  or smoked paprika

1/4 teaspoon sea salt

In a food processor, pulse the garlic and jalapeño until finely chopped. Add the oil, Aleppo pepper, Urfa biber, and salt and process until smooth. Keep in an airtight container in the refrigerator for up to 5 days.

TIP

If you'd like to save time, you can substitute for chimichurri or the zhoug on page 55, if you have it on hand already.

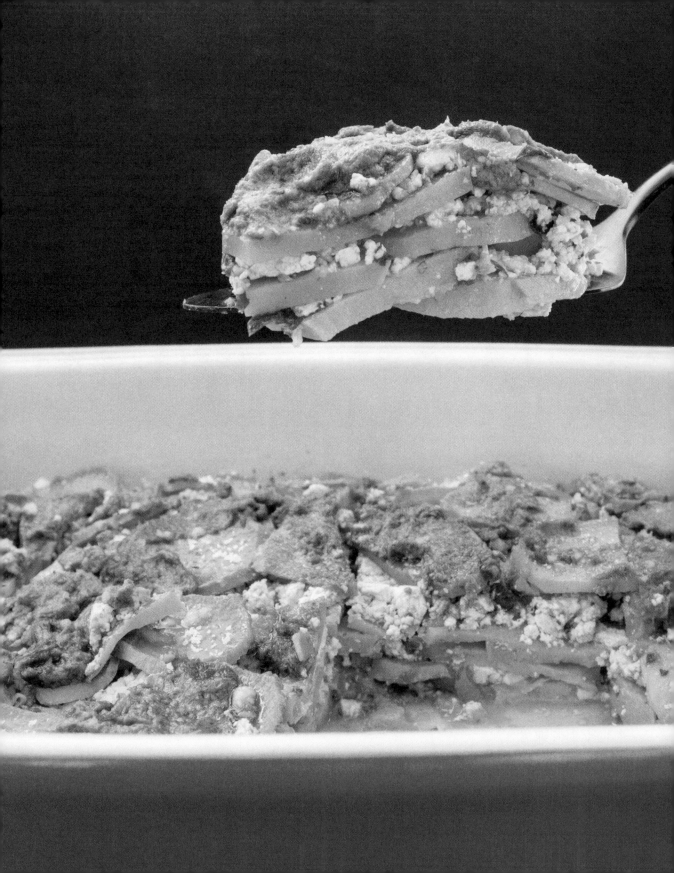

SWEET POTATO LASAGNA

SERVES 2 TO 4   **PREP TIME 20 MIN**   **COOKING TIME 1 HR**   **TOTAL TIME 1 HR 20 MIN**

When I was first evolving vegan, my mom asked me what she could cook me for Easter dinner. At this point, I was still slowly cutting out animal products from my diet and was having the occasional dairy products. I told her I would have her béchamel if she didn't add the usual ground beef in it and she almost laughed at me. That night, all I ate was rice, and 10 minutes into dinner, she started crying because she didn't have anything for me to eat. You see, she thought I was bluffing and that I would cave-in and eat all her wonderful food. Ever since then, she cooks me all her vegan recipes when I come home, but I will never forget that moment. So, I wanted to come up with a lasagna dish that I could cook for every celebratory meal. And this one is a winner. The sweet potatoes stand in for the typical noodle, and instead of béchamel sauce or cheese, there is tofu ricotta. To top it all off, I use a homemade pesto that is simple but delicious! The next time your mom refuses to make her lasagna vegan, you have one from yours truly.

¼ cup extra-virgin olive oil, plus more for greasing

⅓ cup freshly squeezed lemon juice (from about 2 lemons)

12 ounces extra-firm tofu, drained and crumbled

3 tablespoons nutritional yeast

½ cup loosely packed fresh basil leaves

1 tablespoon dried oregano

¼ cup cashews

Sea salt and freshly ground black pepper

3 sweet potatoes, thinly sliced lengthwise ⅛ inch thick

FOR THE PESTO

1 cup packed fresh basil leaves, finely chopped

2 garlic cloves, peeled

¼ cup pine nuts

¼ cup shredded vegan parmesan cheese

½ cup olive oil

Sea salt and freshly ground black pepper

1. Preheat the oven to 375°F with a rack in the upper third. Lightly grease a 9 by 13-inch baking dish with oil.

2. In a food processor, combine the olive oil, lemon juice, tofu, nutritional yeast, basil, oregano, and cashews. Season with salt and pepper and pulse until the ingredients become a grainy puree (like ricotta cheese). Transfer the tofu mixture to a bowl and set aside. Rinse the food processor bowl and blade.

3. Use some of the sweet potato slices to cover the bottom of the prepared baking dish, allowing the slices to overlap slightly and forming an even layer. Spoon one-third of the tofu mixture over the sweet potatoes. Repeat to make another layer of sweet potatoes, top with the remaining tofu mixture, and finish with a third layer of sweet potatoes. Cover tightly with aluminum foil and bake on the top rack until the sweet potatoes are tender when pierced with the tip of a knife, about 50 minutes.

4. Meanwhile, make the pesto: In a food processor, combine the basil, garlic, pine nuts, and parmesan. Pulse a few times to coarsely chop everything. With the food processor running, slowly drizzle in the olive oil. Season with salt and pepper and process until the pesto is smooth adding water 1 tablespoon at a time as needed to thin the sauce to your desired consistency.

5. Remove the lasagna from the oven and discard the foil. Switch the oven to broil. Broil the lasagna on the top rack until the top layer of sweet potatoes is browned in spots, 2 to 4 minutes (keep a careful eye on the lasagna, as broiler heats vary and you don't want it to burn).

6. Serve the lasagna drizzled with the pesto.

TIP

If you really want to take your lasagna to the next level, trim each slice of sweet potato into a rectangle for a more traditional presentation.

PASTA & "MEATBALLS"

SERVES 2   **PREP TIME 15 MIN**   **COOKING TIME ABOUT 25 MIN**   **TOTAL TIME 40 MIN**

I don't think there's anything else in this world that brings us all closer together than pasta and meatballs. Much like pizza, this dish made its way from Italy onto all of our childhood dining tables. Whenever my mom didn't have much time to cook us dinner, we would get a heaping serving of spaghetti and meatballs. And with all the different kinds of pasta now made from chickpeas, corn, and lentils, I think we all should have a go-to recipe for pasta and "meatballs." The secret to this dish is the meatless ground "beef" you use: there are some brands that can be a little too sweet for my liking. And like any childhood classic, don't be afraid to play around with this until you get it just like Mom used to make!

FOR THE TOMATO SAUCE

2 tablespoons olive oil

1 small yellow onion, chopped

2 garlic cloves, finely chopped

1/2 jalapeño, finely chopped

1 (28-ounce) can crushed tomatoes

Sea salt

FOR THE "MEATBALLS"

12 ounces plant-based ground "beef," such as Beyond Beef, Impossible, or Lightlife

1 small red onion, grated

2 garlic cloves, finely chopped

1/2 cup bread crumbs (regular or gluten-free)

2 teaspoons ground cumin

2 teaspoons paprika

1 1/2 teaspoons chili powder

1 1/2 teaspoons ground coriander

2 tablespoons olive oil

TO SERVE

12 ounces of your favorite dried pasta

Fresh basil leaves, for garnish (optional)

1   Bring a large pot of salted water to a boil.

2   Make the tomato sauce: In a large skillet, heat the olive oil over medium-high heat. Add the onion, garlic, and jalapeño and cook until softened and lightly golden, 2 to 3 minutes. Add the tomatoes and season with salt. Bring to a boil. Reduce the heat to medium-low and simmer while you prepare the meatballs.

3   Make the meatballs: In a large bowl, combine the ground "beef," onion, garlic, bread crumbs, cumin, paprika, chili powder, coriander, and 1 tablespoon of the olive oil. Using a fork or your hands, mix until well combined. Form the mixture into 8 balls.

4   In a medium nonstick skillet, heat the remaining 1 tablespoon oil over medium-high heat. Add the meatballs and cook, turning occasionally, until browned all over, 4 to 5 minutes (they may not be cooked through but will finish cooking in the sauce). Transfer the meatballs to the skillet with the sauce and simmer for about 15 minutes.

5   Meanwhile, add the pasta to the boiling water and cook according to the package directions, then drain.

6   Divide the pasta between two bowls. Top with the meatballs and sauce, garnish with fresh basil, if desired, and serve.

TIP

If you don't want to mix your sauce and meatballs, you can cook the meatballs in the oven after searing them in the pan!

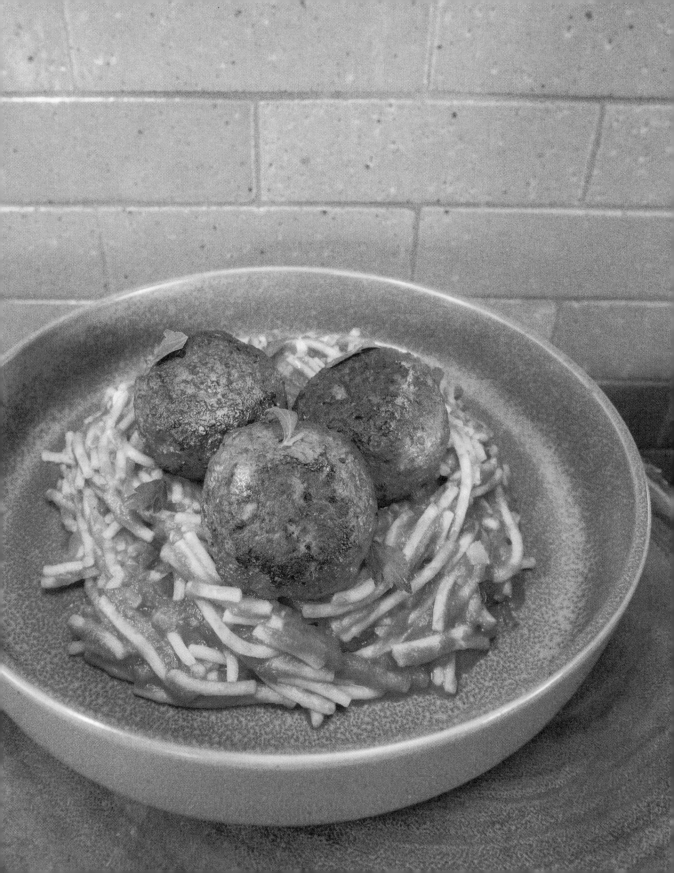

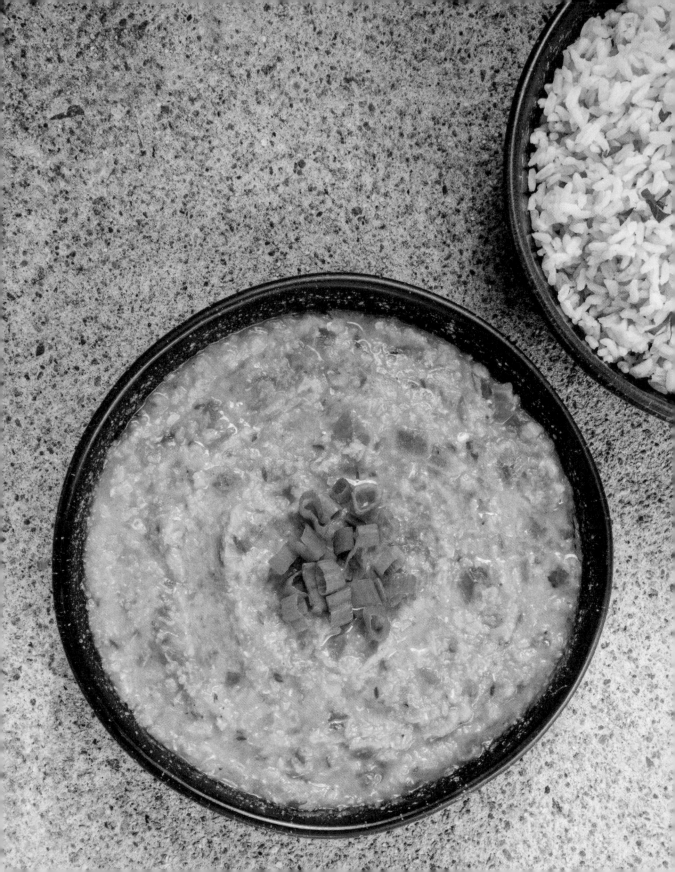

RED LENTIL DAL

SERVES **4**   PREP TIME **5 TO 7 MIN**   COOKING TIME **22 TO 27 MIN**   TOTAL TIME **27 TO 34 MIN**

As I've already mentioned, I love Indian food. I first came up with this recipe after living in London for seven months. London is the capital of Indian cuisine in Europe, so I wanted to eat as much of it as possible! And after having my fair share of dal, I noticed it was actually a pretty simple dish to make. I continue to play with this recipe, but this rendition is a good starting point for anyone cooking Indian food for the first time. It's got some essential ingredients found in Indian cuisine like cumin seeds and ginger, which are simple but flavorful. You can serve this with a side of naan or—my preference for this particular dish—jasmine rice. Either way, this recipe will get you hooked on Indian cuisine!

1 cup dried split red lentils, rinsed

2 plum tomatoes

2 tablespoons coconut oil

1 tablespoon cumin seeds

1 small red onion, diced

1 ½ teaspoons finely chopped fresh ginger

2 garlic cloves, finely chopped

1 teaspoon finely chopped serrano pepper (from about ½ pepper)

1 ½ teaspoons chili powder

Sea salt and freshly ground black pepper

Steamed brown jasmine rice, for serving

Lime wedges, for serving

1   In a large pot, combine the lentils and 3 cups water. Bring to a boil over high heat, then reduce the heat to medium and simmer until the lentils are very soft and the water has been mostly absorbed, 20 to 25 minutes (keep an eye on the water and add more as needed until the lentils are cooked through).

2   Meanwhile, grate the tomatoes into a bowl. Set aside.

3   In a medium skillet, melt the coconut oil over medium heat. Add the cumin and cook until fragrant and lightly toasted, about 1 minute. Add the onion, ginger, garlic, and serrano. Cook, stirring occasionally, until the onion is softened and lightly golden, 1 to 2 minutes.

4   Add the grated tomato and any juices from the bowl and bring to a boil. Add the lentils and reduce the heat to medium-low. Stir in the chili powder and season with salt and black pepper.

5   Serve with jasmine rice and lime wedges for squeezing over.

SPICY DAN DAN NOODLES

SERVES 4   **PREP TIME 10 MIN**   **COOKING TIME 20 TO 25 MIN**   **TOTAL TIME 30 TO 35 MIN**

I love traveling for food because sometimes the most unlikely places are where you find hidden gems. When my producing partners first told me we were going to stop in Washington, DC, as part of our tour, I looked at them like they were crazy. DC isn't known for its vegan community, and I had never heard of a single popular plant-based restaurant there. Yet Fancy Radish was one of many surprising stops in DC, and their food was on fire! And I don't just mean spicy. Their food seemed so simple, but the layers of flavor blew me away. This dish in particular resonated with me and truly made an impression. The creaminess of the tahini combined with the different oils in the sauce is magnificent. Pair it with perfectly cooked noodles and baked shiitake mushrooms, and this dish feels like something you would try on the streets of Thailand or Japan. If you don't like mushrooms, have it without or sub another vegetable—the secret is the sauce!

Sea salt

1 tablespoon balsamic vinegar

3 tablespoons sesame oil

1 garlic clove, finely chopped

1 teaspoon finely chopped
 fresh ginger

1 teaspoon Chinese five-spice
 powder

1 teaspoon tamari

10 ounces shiitake mushroom
 caps, sliced into thin strips

6 ounces uncooked chuka
 soba noodles

2 teaspoons safflower oil

FOR THE DAN DAN SAUCE

1/4 cup sriracha

1/4 cup tahini

1/4 cup tamari

1/4 teaspoon freshly ground
 black pepper

1 tablespoon sesame oil

1 teaspoon chile oil

1/2 teaspoon red pepper flakes

1 tablespoon cane sugar

3/4 cup vegetable broth

4 scallions, green parts only,
 thinly sliced on angle,
 for serving

1 Preheat the oven to 450°F. Bring a large pot of salted water to a boil.

2 In a medium bowl, whisk together the vinegar, sesame oil, garlic, ginger, five-spice powder, and tamari. Add the shiitakes and toss to combine. Spread the mushrooms in a single layer on a rimmed baking sheet and pour over any marinade remaining in the bowl. Roast until the mushrooms are wilted and crisped around the edges, 8 to 10 minutes.

3 Meanwhile, add the chuka soba noodles to the boiling water and cook according to the package instructions, then drain and return the noodles to the pot. Toss with the safflower oil to prevent the noodles from sticking.

4 Make the dan dan sauce: In a blender, combine the sriracha, tahini, tamari, black pepper, sesame oil, chile oil, red pepper flakes, sugar, and broth and blend until smooth. Transfer the dan dan sauce to a large saucepan and heat over medium until warmed through, 2 to 3 minutes.

5 Add the noodles to the pan with the sauce and toss to coat. Using tongs, divide the noodles among four deep bowls. Spoon the sauce over the noodles. Top with the mushrooms and scallions and serve immediately.

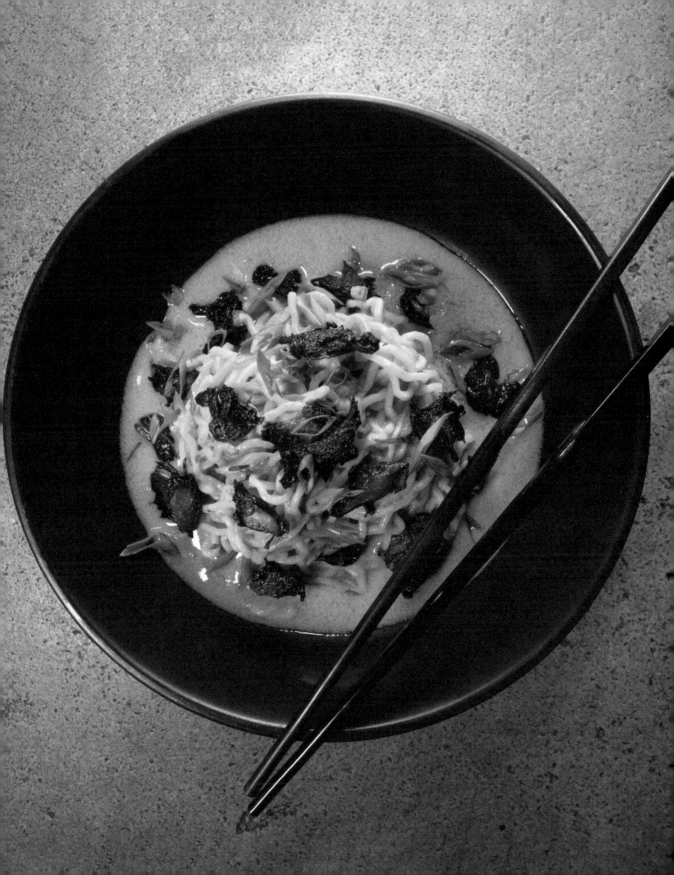

LETTUCE WRAPS WITH SPICY KOREAN BRUSSELS SPROUTS & TOFU

SERVES 2 TO 4   **PREP TIME 20 MIN**   **COOKING TIME 30 MIN**   **TOTAL TIME 50 MIN**

Having worked at a tapas-style restaurant for three years, I know that most people are moving toward communal eating experiences, whether it be for breakfast, lunch, or dinner. Diners want to share their food and try other people's food. Heck, if it weren't so taboo, I'd ask the people at the tables next to me if I could try their food! Even when couples go out to eat, many prefer to order a few dishes to share, react to together, and talk about, learning about each other's palates as they eat. That's why I love this dish. Not only is it packed with flavor and spice and so incredibly light and healthy, but it's made to share. It pairs beautifully with drinks because it's crisp and fresh, but it can also be eaten as a full meal. What I absolutely love about it is that it takes two foods most people raise an eyebrow at—tofu and Brussels sprouts—and transforms them into an interactive dish that will have the whole table clawing for more.

FOR THE GOCHUJANG SAUCE

1 cup packed brown sugar

½ cup rice vinegar

½ cup tamari

½ cup pickled white ginger, drained

½ cup gochujang (Korean red chile paste)

2 tablespoons white miso paste

FOR THE PICKLED CUCUMBERS

1 cucumber, thinly sliced

1 tablespoon white wine vinegar

Pinch of cane sugar

Pinch of sea salt

FOR THE FILLING

1 pound Brussels sprouts, trimmed and halved

4 tablespoons safflower oil

1 (14-ounce) package extra-firm tofu, drained

2 tablespoons sesame seeds

2 romaine hearts, leaves separated, washed, and patted dry

Leaves from 1 bunch cilantro

A few sprigs Thai basil (regular basil will do in a pinch)

½ cup vegan kimchi

1   Preheat the oven to 450°F. Make the gochujang sauce: In a small saucepan, combine the brown sugar, vinegar, and tamari. Cook over medium heat until the sugar has completely dissolved, about 5 minutes, then remove from the heat and transfer to a blender. Add the ginger, gochujang, and miso and blend until smooth. Set aside.

2   Pickle the cucumbers: In a medium bowl, toss together the cucumber slices, vinegar, sugar, and salt. Let marinate while you finish the recipe.

3   Make the filling: On a rimmed baking sheet, toss the Brussels sprouts with 2 tablespoons of the oil and bake until slightly softened and golden, about 15 minutes.

4   Meanwhile, cut the tofu into ½-inch-thick slices and toss with the remaining 2 tablespoons oil. Push the Brussels sprouts to one side of the baking sheet and add the tofu to the other. Bake until the sprouts are tender and browned and the tofu is golden, 10 to 15 minutes.

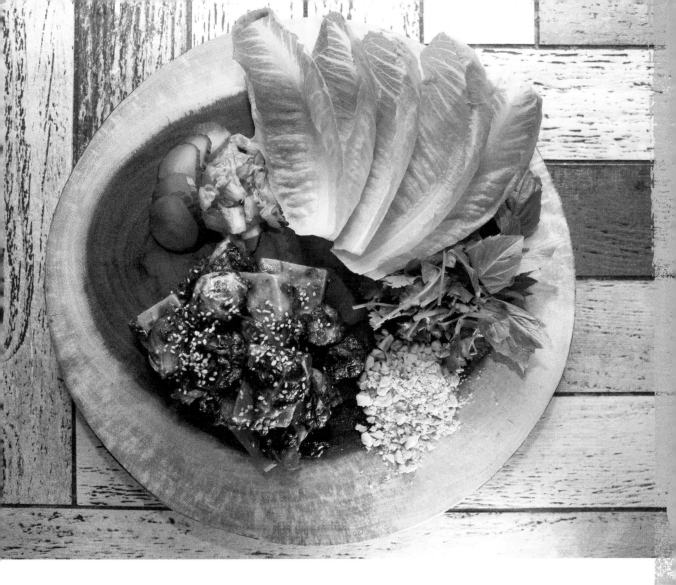

5   In a large bowl, combine the hot Brussels sprouts and tofu with 1 cup of the gochujang sauce (save the rest for another use); toss to coat.

6   Spoon the Brussels sprouts and tofu onto a serving platter. Sprinkle with the sesame seeds. Serve family-style, with the romaine leaves, cilantro, basil, kimchi, and pickled cucumbers in separate dishes alongside, and assemble the wraps at the table.

TIPS

The gochujang sauce can be stored in an airtight container in the fridge overnight or up to one month, if desired—the flavors will keep getting better as it sits.

Vegan kimchi can be found at specialty grocery stores like Whole Foods.

Gochujang, pickled white ginger, and white miso paste can be found at Asian markets and high-end grocery stores like Whole Foods.

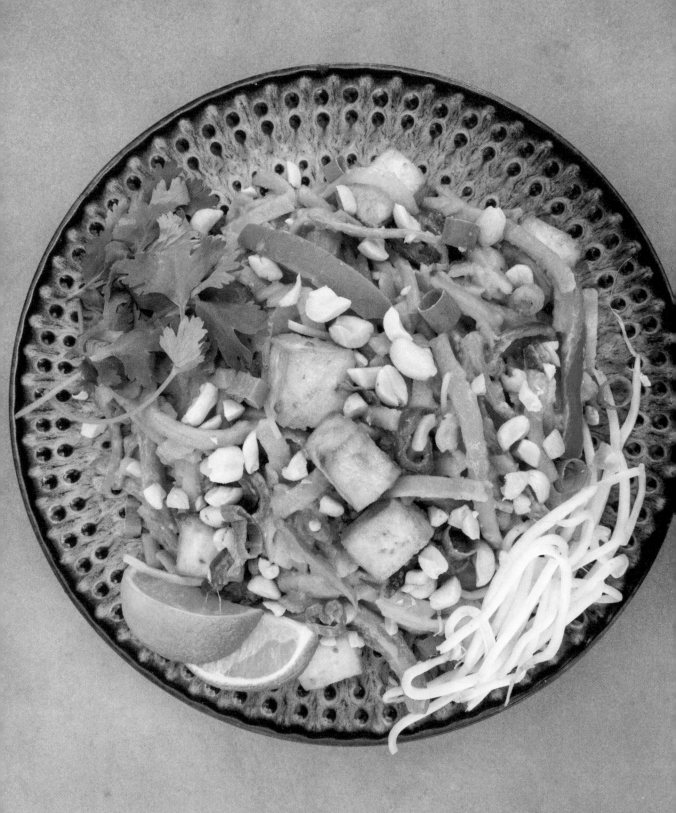

TOFU PAD THAI

SERVES **2 TO 4**   PREP TIME **15 MIN**   COOKING TIME **30 MIN**   TOTAL TIME **45 MIN**

This recipe has a special place in my heart because it's the first one I demonstrated on television. Right before the *Aladdin* press tour, the Hallmark Channel show *Home & Family* invited me on to talk about the film and show their viewers one of my favorite recipes. I wanted to cook something familiar to demonstrate how easy it is to make a dish vegan. All you really have to do with pad thai is take out the eggs and add a plant-based protein. I chose tofu because it's also a great addition to other dishes you can make at home. I make a little extra of this tofu and store it in the fridge for a couple of days to supplement my protein intake. Add it to salads, sandwiches, rice bowls, or eat it on its own! And the kicker is that it's easy and super tasty. I hope you enjoy this tofu pad thai, one of my personal favorites.

FOR THE CRISPY TOFU

1 (14-ounce) block extra-firm tofu, drained and cut into cubes

¼ cup nutritional yeast

1 ½ teaspoons garlic powder

1 tablespoon coconut oil

1 tablespoon tamari

Sea salt and freshly ground black pepper

FOR THE PEANUT SAUCE

¼ cup tamari

1 tablespoon sriracha

1 tablespoon smooth natural peanut butter

FOR THE PAD THAI

8 ounces uncooked Thai brown rice noodles

2 tablespoons coconut oil

1 medium shallot, thinly sliced

2 garlic cloves, thinly sliced

½ jalapeño, thinly sliced

Sea salt and freshly ground black pepper

1 carrot, cut into thin matchsticks

½ red bell pepper, sliced

1 scallion, chopped

Fresh cilantro leaves

2 tablespoons crushed dry-roasted peanuts

Handful of bean sprouts, for serving

Lime wedges, for serving

1   Make the crispy tofu: Preheat the oven to 400°F. In a large bowl, combine the tofu, nutritional yeast, garlic powder, coconut oil, and tamari. Season with salt and pepper and mix well. Sperad the tofu over a rimed baking sheet lined with a silicone baking mat and bake for 30 minutes, flipping halfway through.

2   Meanwhile, make the peanut sauce: In a small bowl, whisk together the tamari, sriracha, and peanut butter until well combined. Set aside.

3   Make the pad thai: Bring a large pot of water to a boil. Add the noodles and cook according to the package directions until al dente. Drain and set aside.

4   In a large skillet, melt the coconut oil over medium-low heat. Add the shallot, garlic, and jalapeño. Season with salt and black pepper and cook until soft. Increase the heat to medium, add the carrot and bell pepper, and cook until lightly browned, about 4 minutes.

5   Add the noodles and sauce to the skillet and mix well. Transfer to a large bowl. Top with the tofu, scallion, cilantro, crushed peanuts, and bean sprouts, and serve with lime wedges for squeezing.

TIPS

The Crispy Tofu can be made in larger batches and used for salads, curries, bowls, and more!

For alternative proteins, you can substitute medium or firm tofu, vegan chick'n, or oyster mushrooms.

PORTL

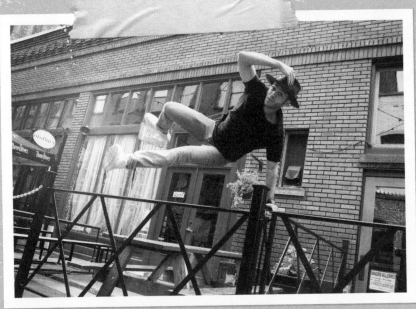

OUT OF ALL THE CITIES WE PLANNED TO VISIT ON OUR EVOLVING VEGAN TOUR, PORTLAND, OREGON, MAY HAVE BEEN THE ONE I WAS MOST EXCITED TO EXPLORE.

I had heard all these stories of how Portland was the fastest-growing vegan scene in North America, and I couldn't wait to see what it was like. The truth is, every city we visited seemed like the fastest-growing to me, but Portland stuck out because of its diverse vegan culture. There was an all-American diner, a vegan Indian café, a plant-based Mediterranean restaurant, and a Taiwanese spot serving up its traditional classics that blew my socks off! The variety and quality here were unmatched for sure. Even in LA, considered the vegan mecca of the world, I'm hard-pressed to find restaurants like the ones we visited in Portland. And the exciting part is, Portland is expanding so rapidly that the possibilities are endless! So yes, if I had to choose one city to go back to strictly for its vegan restaurant scene, it would have to be Portland.

Portland is a beautiful place. We visited during the fall when the leaves were changing colors, and as I took a run around the neighborhood, I found this beautiful trail in the forest. I came to find out later that Portland is home to more than 10,000 acres of preserved nature and public parks! For me, that was the cherry on top. Possibly the most culturally diverse vegan scene in North America, and all this nature to go with it? I'm keeping my fingers crossed that a future job may lead me to live in Portland for a few months. And hopefully it's a role where I have to gain a lot of weight, because, baby, we'd be in business! Next time you're looking for a city to travel to in North America, take a long, hard look at Portland. You won't be disappointed. Oh, and did I mention all the shopping outlets there? Portland—I'll be back!

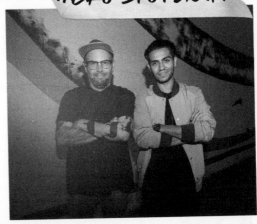

HERO SPOTLIGHT

TAL CASPI
Owner, Aviv

Meeting people like Tal Caspi on this *Evolving Vegan* tour was probably the best part of the whole experience. Food has an incredible power in bringing people together no matter your culture, religion, color, or race, and that's what I love most about the culinary arts. As soon as the crew and I stepped foot into Aviv, Tal's Mediterranean restaurant in Portland, Oregon, he welcomed us with open arms. Tal shares the passion of many of the restaurateurs I had the pleasure of meeting, wanting us to try everything they had on the menu. The drinks, the food, and the ghost pepper ice cream (you read that correctly) just kept on coming! Everything we tried was not only beautiful looking (as you will see in this book) but also beautiful tasting.

The one creation I can't get out of my mind is the ghost pepper ice cream, which had me sweating profusely but it was so addictive, I kept going back for more! It's this creativity and willingness to take risks that really makes Tal a special chef. He takes the rudimentary in the culinary world and puts his own twist on it. It's what makes him and Aviv one of the hottest spots in Portland.

Growing up in an Argentinean household and then working on a goat-dairy farm for years didn't make going vegan easy for Tal. But deep down inside, he says, he always knew that consuming meat products wasn't right for him, even when he was eating and cooking meat for a living. So, a few years ago, Tal teamed up with another restaurateur friend of his—Sanjay Chandrasekaran, owner of The Sudra, which is also featured in this book—and opened up Aviv, where you can treat yourself to the Mediterranean classics like shawarma, labneh, and shakshuka, all made from plants. This spot is so popular in Portland, Tal will never have to milk another goat in his whole life!

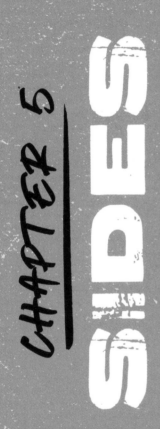

CHAPTER 5
SIDES

Featuring recipes from or inspired by:

AVIV
PORTLAND, OREGON

FANCY RADISH
WASHINGTON, DC

PEÑA PACHAMAMA
SAN FRANCISCO, CALIFORNIA

PURA VITA
LOS ANGELES, CALIFORNIA

RED LENTIL
BOSTON, MASSACHUSETTS

ROSALINDA
TORONTO, CANADA

KALE CHIPS

SERVES 2 OR 3   PREP TIME 10 MIN, PLUS OVERNIGHT SOAKING
COOKING TIME 20 TO 25 MIN   TOTAL TIME 30 TO 35 MIN

As you can imagine, there are certain foods I tried a lot on our tour around North America. One of those is the ever-popular kale chip. I can't remember when I started hearing about kale chips, but after the first time, I never *stopped* hearing about them. The kale chip is easy to get behind as a snack because we all know it's good for us. I mean, after all, it's a dark green leafy vegetable—how can it not be good for us? After a lot of deliberation, I crowned this recipe the best kale chip I tried. One: They're dehydrated, not fried (but as an alternative to buying a very expensive dehydrator, you can bake them in your oven, as I do here). Two: The rub is fantastic! A Bolivian wonder, to say the least.

½ cup cashews, soaked overnight in water to cover, then drained

1 tablespoon freshly squeezed lemon juice

1 tablespoon olive oil

3 tablespoons nutritional yeast

½ teaspoon sea salt

1 bunch curly green kale, stemmed, leaves torn into large pieces

1   Preheat the oven to 300°F with a rack placed in the center of the oven. Line an 11 by 17-inch rimmed baking sheet with parchment paper.

2   In a food processor, combine the cashews, lemon juice, olive oil, nutritional yeast, salt, and 2 tablespoons water. Process until the mixture becomes a mostly smooth, thick paste, drizzling in additional water 1 tablespoon at a time as needed to reach the desired consistency.

3   In a large bowl, combine the kale leaves and cashew paste. Using your hands, rub the leaves to completely coat them with the paste (you want to coat them evenly and avoid any large chunks of paste). Spread the kale in an even layer over the prepared baking sheet.

4   Bake on the center rack, stirring every 5 to 10 minutes, until the kale is dried and crisp, about 25 minutes (keep a close eye on it for those last few minutes, as the kale can go from not done to burnt very quickly at the end). Let cool completely before serving (the chips will crisp up more as they cool).

TIP

Peña Pachamama makes these with Himalayan pink salt, so if you have that on hand, by all means, use it!

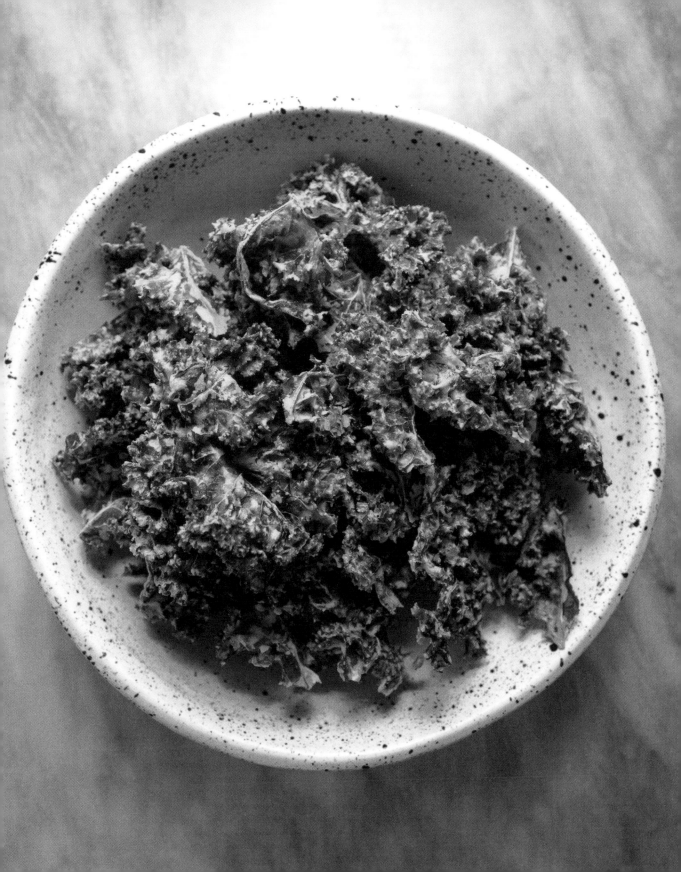

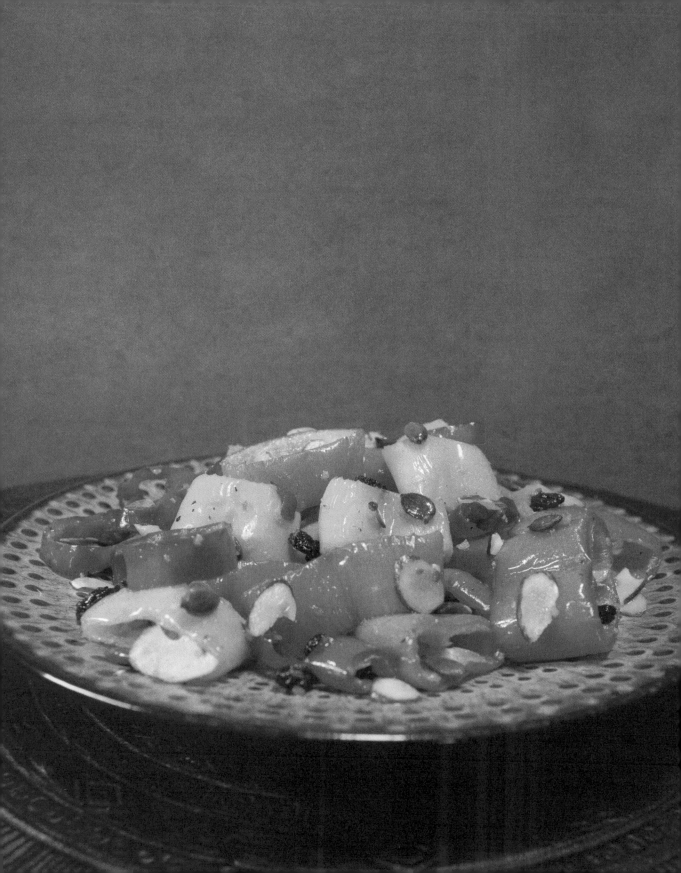

PEPPAS

SERVES 2 TO 4 PREP TIME 10 MIN COOKING TIME 10 TO 15 MIN TOTAL TIME 20 TO 25 MIN

When Pura Vita opened up in West Hollywood, I was the first one in line to try this authentically Italian plant-based restaurant. Do you know how hard it is to find a vegan carbonara or caprese? Damn hard is the answer! Started by chef Tara Punzone, everything in this place screams "Italian"—the wine selection, the food, the vegan gelato. This dish in particular reminds me a lot of my culinary experience in Italy. The combination of the sweet mini peppers and raisins paired with the earthy flavors from the almonds and pumpkin seeds and the spice from the Fresno chile is classic Italian cuisine. This dish is great on its own, as a side, or as an appetizer, and pairs well with almost any wine.

1 pound sweet mini bell peppers, halved crosswise and seeded

½ pound Fresno chiles, seeded and thinly sliced crosswise

3 garlic cloves, finely chopped

2 tablespoons olive oil, plus more for drizzling

2 tablespoons raisins

2 tablespoons pumpkin seeds

2 tablespoons sliced almonds

½ teaspoon red pepper flakes

Sea salt and freshly ground black pepper

1 Preheat the oven to 350°F.

2 In a medium baking dish, toss together the bell peppers, Fresno chiles, garlic, olive oil, raisins, pumpkin seeds, almonds, and red pepper flakes until coated well. Season with salt and black pepper.

3 Bake until the peppers are slightly softened but still have some bite, 10 to 15 minutes. Drizzle with a bit more oil and serve hot or at room temperature.

GRILLED BROCCOLINI WITH CAESAR AIOLI

SERVES 4   PREP TIME 20 MIN   COOKING TIME 15 MIN   TOTAL TIME 35 MIN

Being the youngest of three siblings, I like to learn about vegetables like broccolini because I believe they are often overshadowed, in this case by its older brother, broccoli. Unlike its big brother, broccolini can be cooked whole with its stem because it's far easier to cook through and the whole vegetable absorbs much more flavor than broccoli florets. The stem is also where most of the nutrition is stored, so it's better to eat it than toss it away (as we tend to do with broccoli stems). In this dish, the broccolini is charred using a grill, which gives it that great barbecue flavor we all crave and love, and is served with a caper-onion sauce for a burst of flavor and a vegan Caesar aioli for a creamy and acidic component. This dish is simple, light, and nutritious and has become one of my favorite broccolini recipes of all time. Dig in and conquer your fear of the stem!

3 tablespoons olive oil

1 cup finely chopped white onion (about ½ onion)

Sea salt and freshly ground black pepper

¼ cup capers, rinsed

1 jalapeño, seeded and finely chopped

1 cup vegan mayonnaise

1 tablespoon Dijon mustard

1 teaspoon Tabasco sauce

2 tablespoons vegan Worcestershire sauce

4 garlic cloves, thinly sliced

2 bunches broccolini, cut into 1-inch pieces

1 head baby romaine, quartered, or 10 to 12 small inner leaves from a romaine heart

1 In a large skillet, heat 2 tablespoons of the olive oil over medium heat. Add the onion, season with salt, and cook, stirring occasionally, until softened, about 5 minutes. Remove from the heat. Stir in the capers and as much of the jalapeño as you like. Transfer to a bowl and set aside to cool while you prepare the aioli. Set the skillet aside (no need to rinse it).

2 In a blender, combine the mayonnaise, mustard, Tabasco, Worcestershire sauce, and half the garlic; blend until smooth, then season with salt and pepper.

3 In the skillet you used to cook the onion, heat the remaining 1 tablespoon oil over medium-high heat. Add the broccolini and remaining garlic and season with salt and pepper. Cover and cook until the broccolini is tender and charred in spots, 3 to 4 minutes. Remove from the heat.

4 To serve, spread some of the aioli over individual serving plates (you might have more than you need, so save the rest for another use). Arrange the romaine over the aioli, then top with the broccolini and garlic. Spoon the onion-caper mixture over (again, you may have more than needed, so save the rest for another use) and serve.

TIPS

If you're looking to take the dish even further, here are a couple of great garnishes that really complement it: bread crumbs, crispy onions, or garlic, dill, even pistachios—be bold!

You can also cook this on an outdoor grill.

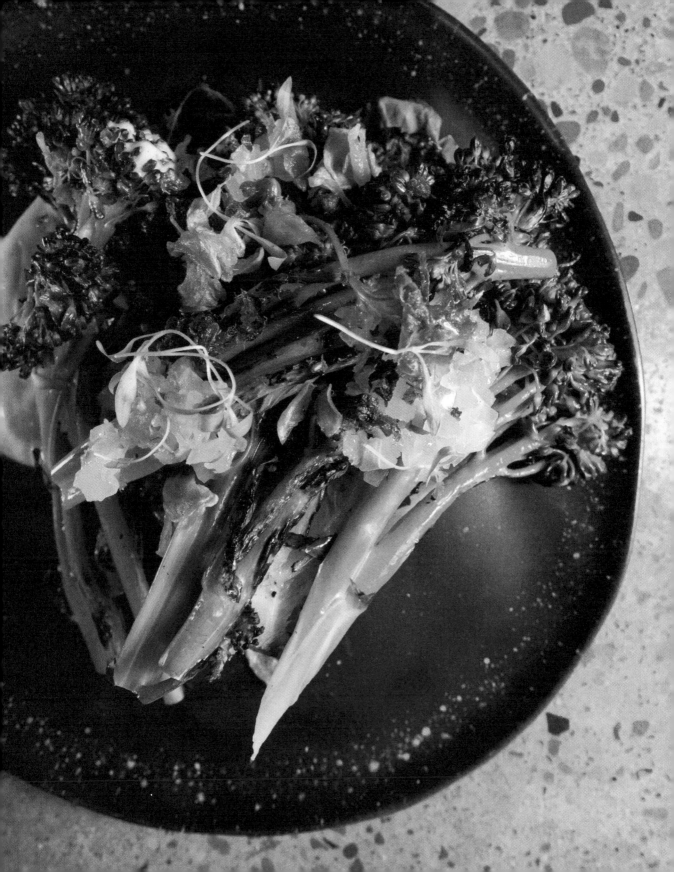

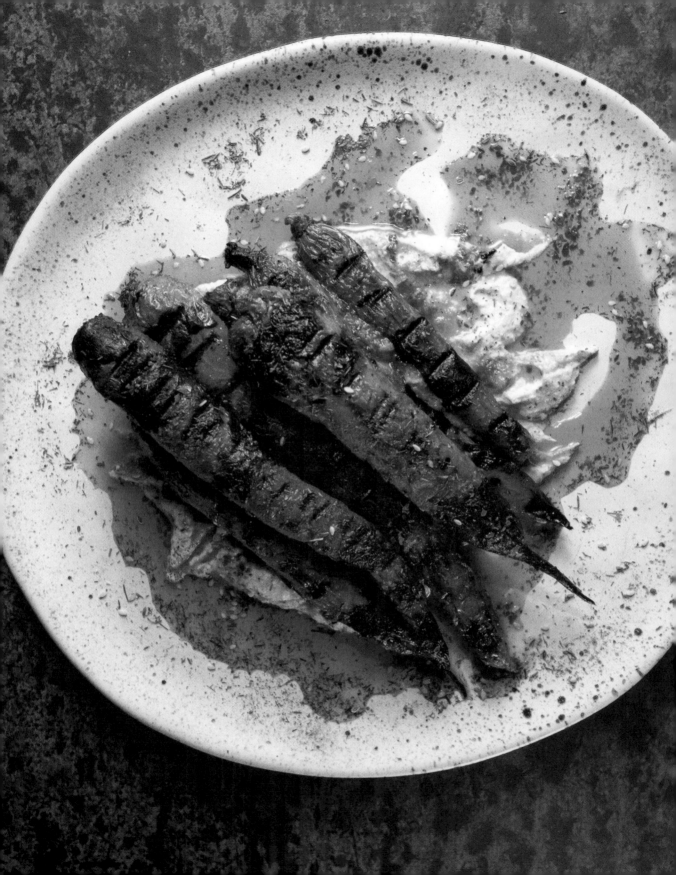

From Aviv in Portland, Oregon

MOROCCAN CARROTS

SERVES 2 **PREP TIME** 5 MIN **COOKING TIME** 60 TO 75 MIN **TOTAL TIME** 65 TO 80 MIN

Anyone who tells me they're going to Portland always gets my recommendation to go visit Aviv. Almost always they come back saying it was one of the best vegan meals they've had. The simple truth is, Tal Caspi, owner and head chef of Aviv, is hella talented and loves food. He's taken a cuisine he loves—Mediterranean cooking—and been incredibly innovative with it. This dish is particularly inspired by his travels to Morocco. He takes such a simple vegetable that we all know—the carrot—and transforms it into a satisfying, creamy, spicy, gorgeous dish (I have to say, the photograph of these carrots is one of my favorite images in this book). What's more, this dish is really not that difficult to make, but I will say this: Do not use store-bought bagged carrots. Go to your local market and pick up the freshest carrots you can find, or at the very least buy the ones from the store that still have their leafy tops attached. It makes all the difference, and you won't regret it.

FOR THE ROASTED CARROTS

6 medium carrots

2 tablespoons olive oil

1 1/2 teaspoons za'atar

1 teaspoon sea salt

FOR THE CASHEW LABNEH

1/2 cup cashews

1/4 cup hot (not boiling) water

2 tablespoons freshly squeezed lemon juice

1/4 teaspoon sea salt

TO SERVE

1 tablespoon olive oil

1 tablespoon harissa paste

Za'atar, for garnish

1 Roast the carrots: Preheat the oven to 300°F.

2 On a rimmed baking sheet, toss the carrots, olive oil, za'atar, and salt. Roast on the center rack until the carrots are just tender (they should still be slightly firm), 60 to 75 minutes.

3 Meanwhile, make the cashew labneh: Combine the cashews, hot water, lemon juice, and salt in a blender. Blend until smooth, adding additional water 1 tablespoon at a time, if needed. (The labneh can be stored in an airtight container in the refrigerator until ready to use, up to 3 days.)

4 When ready to serve, in a small bowl, whisk together the olive oil and harissa paste to combine.

5 Spread the labneh over two serving plates and drizzle the harissa oil over the labneh. Top with the carrots, sprinkle some za'atar over, and serve.

ORANGE CAULIFLOWER BITES

SERVES 2 TO 4   PREP TIME 15 MIN   COOKING TIME 30 TO 35 MIN   TOTAL TIME 45 TO 50 MIN

If you are reading this book, chances are you've eaten some sort of cauliflower appetizer at a restaurant before. Buffalo cauliflower with a ranch or blue cheeze dressing is all the craze right now, and rightfully so—it's a combination that works. But when I went to Boston and tried these orange cauliflower bites, my palate exploded. I ran around the restaurant cheering and high-fiving people as if I had just discovered water. So, if you thought Buffalo cauliflower was good, just wait until these bad boys come off the pan—things are about to get real exciting.

Sunflower oil, for coating

½ cup chickpea flour or all-purpose flour

½ teaspoon garlic powder

¼ teaspoon sea salt

1 head cauliflower, cut into florets

FOR THE SAUCE

¼ cup tomato paste

½ jalapeño (use less or more, depending on your heat preference)

2 tablespoons molasses

2 teaspoons ground cumin

2 teaspoons ground coriander

2 teaspoons paprika

2 tablespoons tamari

1 teaspoon finely grated fresh ginger

2 tablespoons sunflower oil

1 small yellow onion, diced

1 red or green bell pepper, diced

1 celery stalk, thinly sliced

¼ cup chopped fresh cilantro

1 Preheat the oven to 450°F. Generously brush an 11 by 17-inch rimmed baking sheet with oil.

2 In a large bowl, whisk together the flour, garlic powder, salt, and ½ cup water until smooth. Add the cauliflower to the bowl and toss to coat. Spread the cauliflower over the prepared baking sheet in a single layer. Bake on the center rack until the cauliflower is golden all over, about 20 minutes, flipping once halfway through.

3 Meanwhile, make the sauce: In a food processor, combine the tomato paste, jalapeño, molasses, cumin, coriander, paprika, tamari, ginger, sunflower oil, and 2 tablespoons water. Process until smooth, then transfer to a separate large bowl.

4 Remove the baking sheet from the oven. Add the cauliflower, onion, bell pepper, and celery to the bowl with the sauce and toss to coat. Spread the vegetables over the baking sheet in a single layer. Bake, stirring occasionally, until the sauce has slightly caramelized and the bell pepper, onion, and celery are softened, 10 to 15 minutes.

5 Spoon the vegetables onto a serving platter. Sprinkle with the cilantro and serve immediately.

TIP

Lining the baking sheet with aluminum foil makes for easier cleanup!

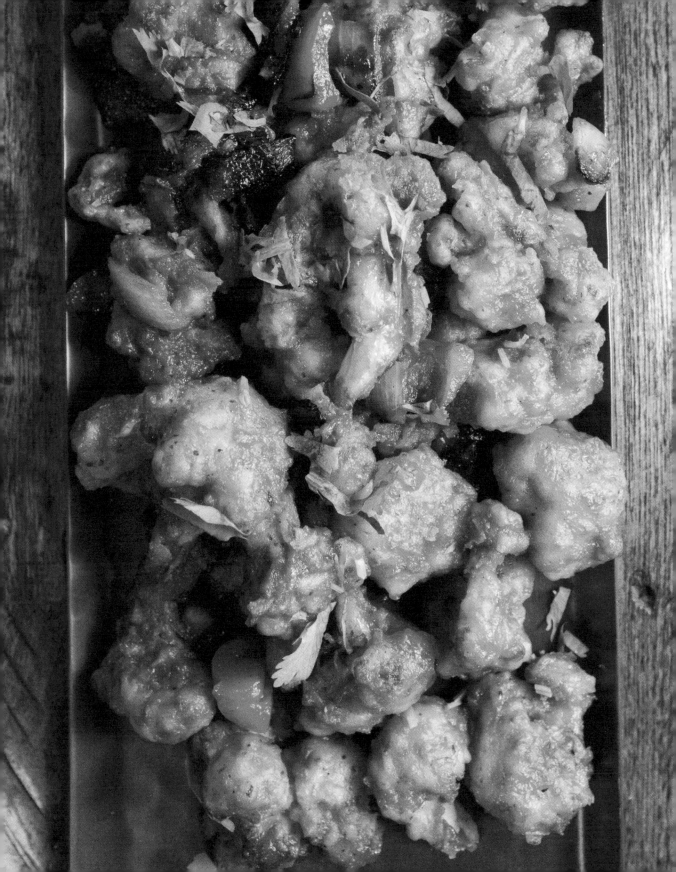

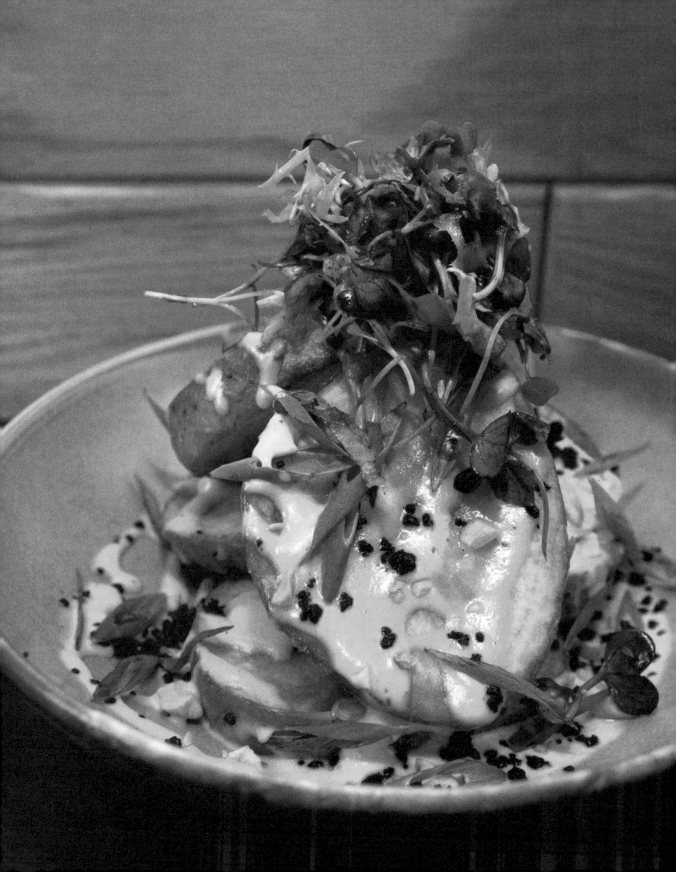

PERUVIAN POTATOES

SERVES 2 TO 4   PREP TIME 10 MIN   COOKING TIME 60 MIN   TOTAL TIME 1 HR 10 MIN

The only thing I like better than a potato is a potato covered in creamy goodness. Now, don't get me wrong—I'm not talking about a creamy potato like a mashed potato. I mean a thick, crisp, baked potato covered in a sauce so creamy, you'll think you died drowning in coconuts (who wouldn't wanna die drowning in a coconut, amirighttt?!). These Peruvian potatoes from Fancy Radish, one of my favorite restaurants from our tour, are baked to perfection, drizzled with a velvety sauce, and topped with scallions, olives, and roasted peanuts. What more can I say? There may just be a perfect potato after all.

2 large russet potatoes

Sea salt

FOR THE AJÍ AMARILLO SAUCE

¼ cup ají amarillo paste

½ cup vegan mayonnaise

1 garlic clove, peeled

1 teaspoon finely chopped shallot

1 tablespoon olive oil

1 ½ teaspoons freshly squeezed lime juice

Pinch of ground cumin

Sea salt and freshly ground black pepper

TO SERVE

Sunflower or peanut oil, for frying

2 tablespoons chopped roasted salted peanuts

2 tablespoons finely chopped pitted oil-cured black olives

1 scallion, thinly sliced

1 tablespoon chopped fresh cilantro

Handful of microgreens

1 Preheat the oven to 450°F.

2 Pierce the potatoes a few times with the tip of a paring knife, season with salt, then wrap each individually in aluminum foil. Bake until tender and easily pierced with a fork, about 45 minutes. Remove from the foil and let cool completely.

3 Meanwhile, make the ají amarillo sauce: In a blender, combine the ají amarillo paste, mayonnaise, garlic, shallot, olive oil, lime juice, and cumin. Blend until smooth; season with salt and pepper.

4 Once the potatoes are cool, cut them crosswise into ¼-inch-thick slices.

5 Fill a large skillet with ¼ inch of oil and heat the oil over medium-high heat until shimmering. Add the potato slices, in batches as needed to avoid overcrowding the pan, and cook, flipping once, until golden brown, about 2 minutes per side. Transfer to the prepared plate to drain.

6 Divide the potatoes among individual serving plates, drizzle with the ají amarillo sauce, and garnish with the peanuts, olives, scallion, cilantro, and microgreens. Serve immediately.

TORON

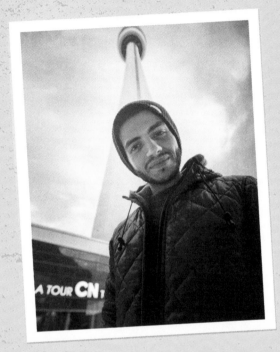

AH, YES. THE CITY I STILL CALL HOME.

After immigrating to Canada when I was three years old, I lived in Toronto and its surrounding suburbs for more than twenty years. My family and I first lived in a neighborhood called Scarborough, which was very ethnically diverse, and even though I was very young, I felt at home there. After a couple of years, we moved to a small suburb called Markham, which, many years later, isn't very small anymore! Markham wasn't as culturally diverse at the time, but it's where I grew up and went to high school. My parents were very resistant to my dropping out of the University of Toronto, where I was studying neuroscience, to transfer to an acting program

at "some place called Ryerson," but I stuck to my guns. With that transfer also came a move to downtown Toronto. It was there that I think I went from being a teenager to an adult and enjoyed some of the best years of my life thus far. When I finally graduated from theater school, I started looking into veganism.

My two best friends, Eddie (who I was living with at the time) and Josh (who I lived with the year prior), and I started doing our research into how meat consumption affected our health and the planet. And not to mention the animal cruelty involved, which was horrifying, to say the least. Together, we slowly encouraged each other to evolve vegan. And with money finally coming in, some from acting but mostly from my restaurant job, I started to go out and explore vegan cuisine. I remember the first time Eddie and I tried superfood, vegan, gluten-free muffins from a local bakery called Bunner's Bakeshop—our minds were blown! We went back weekly to buy half a dozen muffins each. And with this evolving lifestyle,

TO

we also began to hit the gym hard! We realized that plant-based eating didn't just support our workouts; it actually made us feel lighter, more energetic, and stronger. We started seeing bodily transformations we had never seen before, and we associated much of those to our changing diet.

Everyone always asks me, "When did you go vegan?" And the truth is, it's hard to answer that question, because I truly did evolve toward a plant-based lifestyle slowly; it was never an overnight decision. But one day does stand out in my memory: Eddie, Josh, and I went to the Dundas Escarpment, an hour outside Toronto, hiked to a small waterfall, and had a vegan picnic. I recall thinking, *If being out in nature and discussing life and friendships is what it means to be vegan, then count me in.*

Toronto will always be home to me because I spent some of my most formative years there, and I'm happy to know that the city's vegan scene continues to evolve rapidly. Toronto: thank you for preparing me for life. I will always call you home.

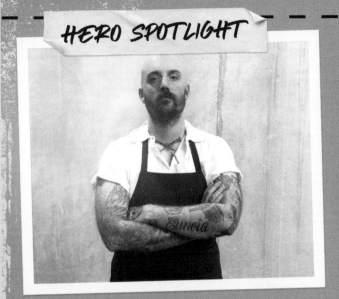

HERO SPOTLIGHT

MATTHEW RAVENSCROFT
Head Chef, Rosalinda

Matthew Ravenscroft, head chef of the Mexican restaurant Rosalinda in downtown Toronto, is one of those people you might see on the streets and immediately be drawn to. He's six-foot-something, with tattoos all over, and wears a big ginger beard. Once you start talking with him, you come to the conclusion that he's as approachable and nice as you would want someone to be. Chef Ravenscroft has a different approach when it comes to veganism. He says that instead of focusing on the politics of it all (and trust me, there is a lot of politics involved), his mission at the restaurant is all about "creating a great experience that's tailored to people's needs." In other words, it's all about cooking great food made from plants. It's that simple. When I asked him why vegan Mexican food and why now, he explained that it's one of those cuisines that naturally lends itself to a plant-based experience. Historically, Mexicans eat a lot of vegan food, and people who can't afford meat or fish naturally eat mostly vegan anyways.

Now, let's be clear. This is not the same Mexican restaurant where I waited tables for over three years. Back in 2014, there was no vegan Mexican restaurant in Toronto. In fact, plant-based establishments weren't really a part of the culture in Toronto the way they are now! Today, a place like Rosalinda is packed every night of the week! Vegan restaurants in metropolitan cities like Toronto and New York are all the rave—and they have the game to back it up. The food here is delicious, the ambience is delightful, and the people running the operation, Matthew included, are incredibly dedicated. Right now in Toronto, there doesn't seem to be anything hotter than a new plant-based restaurant, like Rosalinda.

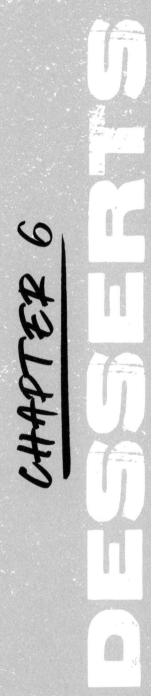

CHAPTER 6
DESSERTS

Featuring recipes from or inspired by:

FOMU ICE CREAM
BOSTON, MASSACHUSETTS

INDIGO AGE CAFE
VANCOUVER, CANADA

LITTLE CHOC APOTHECARY
BROOKLYN, NEW YORK

MAMMA'S KITCHEN

PEACE PIES
SAN DIEGO, CALIFORNIA

ROSALINDA
TORONTO, CANADA

STICKY FINGERS SWEETS & EATS
WASHINGTON, DC

SWEET HART KITCHEN
TORONTO, CANADA

TRILOGY SANCTUARY
SAN DIEGO, CALIFORNIA

VEGGIE GALAXY
CAMBRIDGE, MASSACHUSETTS

From Sticky Fingers Sweets & Eats in Washington, DC

APPLE PIE

SERVES **8**   PREP TIME **25 MIN**   COOKING TIME **45 MIN**   TOTAL TIME **1 HR 10 MIN**

I don't know about you, but whenever I hear "pie," I think two things: *delicious* and *pain in the ass*. Let's be honest—baking a pie from scratch sounds just as hard as brain surgery, and the most intimidating part is making the crust. If that's going to prevent you from trying this recipe, I recommend finding a ready-made vegan pie crust and moving straight to the filling. Of course, my preference is that you challenge yourself and try making the crust using this recipe. Especially because it's a recipe from Doron Petersan, a two-time *Cupcake Wars* champion! And just like with Doron's muffin recipe on page 24, feel free to get creative and try different fillings. Peach, strawberry, and blueberry are always good options, but you can't really go wrong—just make sure whatever fruit you use has some moisture in it.

FOR THE PIE CRUST

1 cup all-purpose flour, plus more for dusting

1 teaspoon cane sugar

Pinch of sea salt

6 tablespoons very cold vegan butter, cut into chunks

1 teaspoon apple cider vinegar

2 tablespoons ice-cold water

FOR THE CRUMB TOPPING

1 cup all-purpose flour

1/3 cup packed dark brown sugar

Pinch of sea salt

6 tablespoons vegan butter, melted

FOR THE FILLING

6 to 8 apples (about 2 pounds), peeled, cored, and thinly sliced

3/4 cup cane sugar

1/4 cup all-purpose flour

1 1/2 teaspoons ground cinnamon

1 teaspoon ground nutmeg

Pinch of sea salt

1   Preheat the oven to 425°F with a rack placed in the lower third.

2   Make the pie crust: In a food processor, combine the flour, sugar, and salt. Pulse to blend. Add the butter and pulse a few times just until it forms a crumbly mixture with some pea-size pieces. Add the vinegar and cold water. Pulse just until the dough comes together. Scrape the dough onto a lightly floured counter. Knead once or twice and form the dough into a 1-inch-thick disc.

3   Sprinkle a little more flour on the counter, then roll the dough into a 13-inch round. Transfer it to a 9-inch metal pie pan (do not use a glass, ceramic, or deep-dish plate), pressing gently to fit the dough into the pan. Crimp the edges and chill in the refrigerator.

4   Make the crumb topping: In a medium bowl, whisk together the flour, brown sugar, and salt. Add the melted butter and stir with a fork until blended and there are no visible traces of flour. Set aside.

5   Make the filling: In a large bowl, combine the apples, sugar, flour, cinnamon, nutmeg, and salt. Toss to coat.

6   Transfer the apple filling to the chilled pie crust, scraping any juices from the bowl over the apples. Evenly sprinkle the crumb topping over the filling. Bake on the bottom rack for 15 minutes.

7   Reduce the oven temperature to 350°F and bake until the filling begins to bubble and the apples are tender when pierced with the tip of a paring knife, about 30 minutes. If the topping or edges of the crust begin to brown too quickly, cover the pie loosely with a piece of aluminum foil. Transfer the pie to a wire rack and let cool completely before serving.

TIP

Using a mix of apple varieties is good for flavor and texture—I used Granny Smith, Jonah gold, and McIntosh.

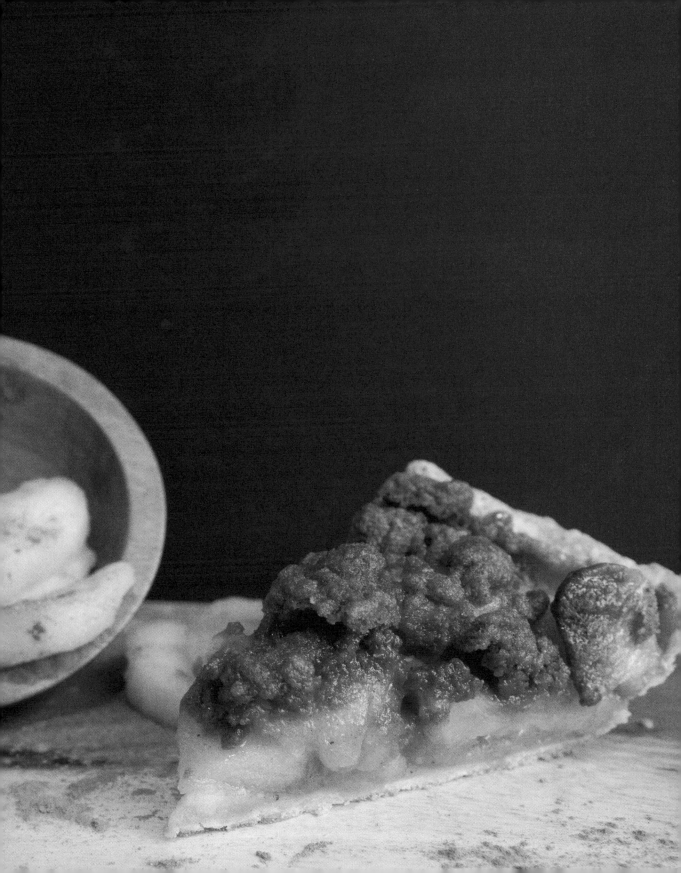

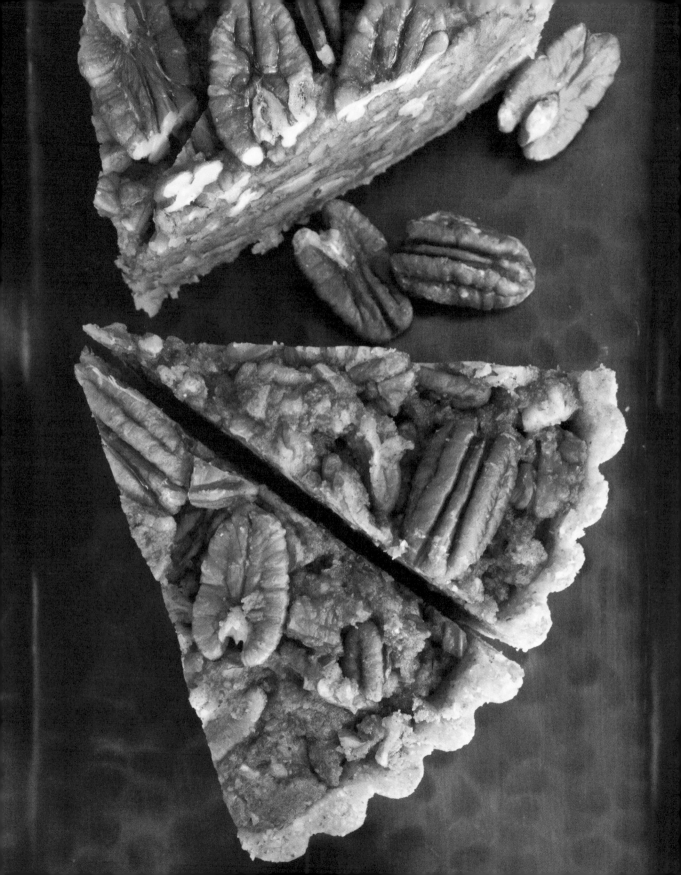

NO-BAKE MAPLE PECAN PIE

SERVES **8 TO 10**   PREP TIME **30 MIN**   SETTING TIME **30 TO 60 MIN**   TOTAL TIME **60 TO 90 MIN**

I first met Alexandra, the owner of Sweet Hart Kitchen, back in Toronto at a small vegan food fair. At the time, Alex was building her brand, doing pop-ups in the city and operating out of a commercial kitchen fulfilling orders that she received through family and friends. It was truly love at first bite when I tried her Snickers-inspired mini bars at the fair. They were raw, gluten-free, and made from only a couple of ingredients, and tasted exactly like my favorite chocolate bar growing up. I knew she was going to do great things, because not only was she a sweetheart (no pun intended), she was one hell of a talented chef! When she first opened Sweet Hart Kitchen in Kensington Market, one of the most famous markets in Canada, everything she offered was not only vegan and gluten-free but also raw. She has since started offering baked goods at the shop, but this recipe is an homage to her early days: a no-bake, completely raw, fully vegan, and gluten-free pecan pie.

FOR THE CRUST

3 cups almond flour

2 cups unsweetened shredded coconut

1 cup pure maple syrup

½ cup smooth natural almond butter, well stirred

½ teaspoon ground cinnamon

½ teaspoon sea salt

FOR THE FILLING

1 cup Medjool dates, pitted

½ cup coconut oil, melted

1 ½ teaspoons pure vanilla extract

½ teaspoon sea salt

½ cup warm (not hot or boiling) water

1 cup almond flour

1 cup chopped raw pecans, plus ¾ cup pecan halves for topping

¼ cup plus 1 tablespoon pure maple syrup

2 teaspoons pumpkin pie spice

1   Make the crust: Line an 8-inch round tart pan with a removable bottom with parchment paper (it's okay if the paper comes slightly over the edge of the pan).

2   In a food processor, combine the almond flour, shredded coconut, maple syrup, almond butter, cinnamon, and salt. Pulse until the dough comes together and forms a ball. Press the dough over the bottom and up the sides of the prepared tart pan. Refrigerate while you prepare the filling.

3   Make the filling: Wipe the food processor bowl and blade clean. Place the dates, coconut oil, vanilla, and salt in the food processor. With the food processor running, slowly pour in the warm water (you may not need to use it all) until the mixture is very smooth and caramel-like. Transfer the date caramel to a large bowl.

4   Add the almond flour, chopped pecans, ¼ cup of the maple syrup, and the pumpkin pie spice to the bowl with the date caramel. Stir with a wooden spoon until well combined, with no visible almond flour (the filling will be stiff; if you have a stand mixer with the paddle attachment, it will make this part easier).

5   Scrape the filling into the chilled crust. Use a lightly greased spatula or your fingers to smooth the filling out evenly to the edges of the pan.

6   In a medium bowl, toss the pecan halves with the remaining 1 tablespoon maple syrup until well coated. Press the pecans into the top of the filling. Refrigerate the pie for 1 hour or freeze for 30 minutes before serving.

BASBOUSA (COCONUT CRUMBLE CAKE)

SERVES **6 TO 8**   PREP TIME **15 MIN**   COOKING TIME **40 MIN**   TOTAL TIME **55 MIN**

I didn't get to spend much time with my grandmother when I was a kid because she lived in Egypt and I grew up in Canada. But there are a few things I remember very fondly about her. She loved—and I mean *loved—basbousa* paired with a warm tea latte. She was a simple woman, but those two things got her Egyptian blood flowing heavy in her veins, both figuratively and literally (she had very high cholesterol). This cake made me crazy when I was a kid, too. Any time my dad and I heard my mom was baking *basbousa*, we would plan the whole day around it. We made sure we stocked up on mint and tea—because as my grandmother knew, nothing pairs better with *basbousa* than a hot cup of tea—we avoided pissing Mom off the whole day so she could concentrate, and we definitely left room for dessert after dinner so we could have a slice or two. Or three. Or . . . you know what? We ate the whole cake, okay?!

FOR THE CAKE

- **1/3 cup coconut oil, melted, plus more for greasing**
- **1 1/4 cups well-shaken canned coconut milk**
- **1/2 cup cane sugar**
- **1 1/2 cups semolina**
- **1 cup unsweetened finely shredded desiccated coconut**
- **1 teaspoon baking powder**
- **1 teaspoon pure vanilla extract**
- **1/2 cup blanched almonds, split in half**

FOR THE SYRUP

- **1 1/2 cups cane sugar**
- **1 teaspoon freshly squeezed lemon juice**

1. Make the cake: Preheat the oven to 375°F. Lightly grease the bottom and sides of an 8-inch square baking dish with coconut oil.

2. In a large bowl, whisk together the melted coconut oil, coconut milk, and sugar. Add the semolina, shredded coconut, baking powder, and vanilla and gently stir until just combined.

3. Scrape the batter into the prepared baking dish, spreading it out evenly in the pan. Using a sharp knife, score the top of the batter into 1-inch pieces. Place a couple of almonds, split-side down, onto each scored section.

4. Bake until golden brown and a skewer inserted into the center comes out mostly clean, 35 to 40 minutes.

5. Meanwhile, make the syrup: In a small saucepan, combine the sugar and 1 1/2 cups water. Bring to a boil over medium-high heat and cook until the sugar has completely dissolved, 2 to 3 minutes. Remove from heat, stir in the lemon juice, and keep warm.

6. When the cake is ready, remove it from the oven and cut it along the scored lines (do not remove the pieces from the pan yet). Pour the warm syrup over the hot cake. Let the cake cool completely in the pan before serving.

TIP

Start the homemade syrup once the *basbousa* has gone into the oven, then keep it warm while the cake is baking. This will give you more than enough time to make the syrup.

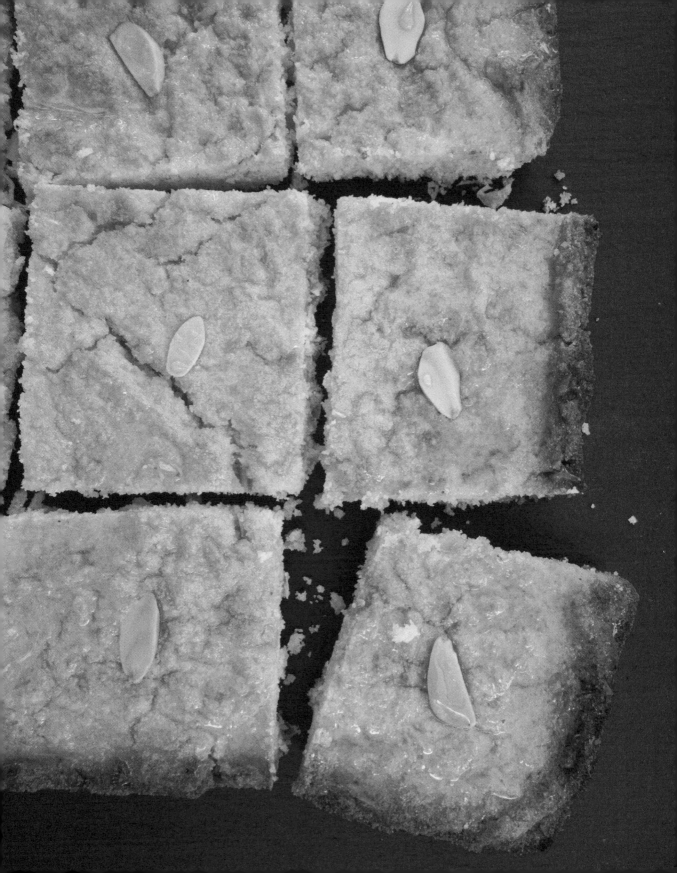

BOSTON CREAM PIE-CAKE

**SERVES 8 TO 10   PREP TIME 20 MIN   COOKING TIME 35 TO 37 MIN
TOTAL TIME ABOUT 1 HR, PLUS 4 HRS CHILLING TIME**

Anyone who knows me well will tell you that I have more of a savory tooth than a sweet one. And I have even less of an interest in cakes. So you can imagine my dismay when I found out that a Boston cream pie (something I was actually really looking forward to eating) was actually a cake—I was duped! Reluctant to try this deceptive cake from Boston, I had a tiny bite when my colleagues ordered it at Veggie Galaxy and I have to say . . . it was pretty damn good! Though definitely not a pie, the texture of this cake was drier and firmer than your average cake and I actually liked that much better. Take two layers of custard (that needs at least 4 hours to chill, so keep that in mind when planning this recipe) and three tiers of sponge cake, top it with a chocolaty coating, and you have a Boston cream pie (that's actually a cake). Inspired by Veggie Galaxy's creation, here's my version of the BCP.

FOR THE VANILLA CUSTARD

½ cup cane sugar

¼ cup cornstarch

Pinch of sea salt

2 cups nondairy milk

2 tablespoons vegan butter, cut into 4 pieces, plus more for greasing

2 teaspoons pure vanilla extract

FOR THE CAKE

3 ¾ cups gluten-free all-purpose flour, plus more for dusting

2 ¼ cups nondairy milk

2 tablespoons apple cider vinegar

1 ¾ cups cane sugar

1 ½ tablespoons baking powder

1 ½ teaspoons baking soda

¾ teaspoon sea salt

¾ cup unsweetened applesauce

6 tablespoons neutral oil, such as grapeseed or safflower

1 tablespoon pure vanilla extract

FOR THE CHOCOLATE GLAZE

5 ounces vegan bittersweet chocolate chips

¼ cup cane sugar

½ teaspoon pure vanilla extract

1 tablespoon brown rice syrup

1. Make the vanilla custard: In a small pot, whisk together the sugar, cornstarch, and salt. Slowly whisk in the milk. Cook over medium-high heat, whisking continuously, until thickened to a puddinglike consistency, about 2 minutes. Remove from the heat and whisk in the butter and vanilla. Cover with a piece of plastic wrap pressed directly against the surface of the pudding (this prevents a skin from forming). Refrigerate until completely chilled, at least 4 hours or up to overnight.

2. Once the custard has cooled, make the cake: Preheat the oven to 350°F with a rack placed in the center position. Grease the bottom and sides of three 8-inch round cake pans with vegan butter, then lightly dust with flour, tapping out any excess. Line the bottom of each pan with a round of parchment paper cut to fit.

3. In a large bowl, whisk together the milk and vinegar; set aside for 5 minutes (it will curdle to form a vegan "buttermilk").

4. In a medium bowl, whisk together the flour, sugar, baking powder, baking soda, and salt.

5. Add the applesauce, oil, and vanilla to the bowl with the milk mixture and whisk to combine.

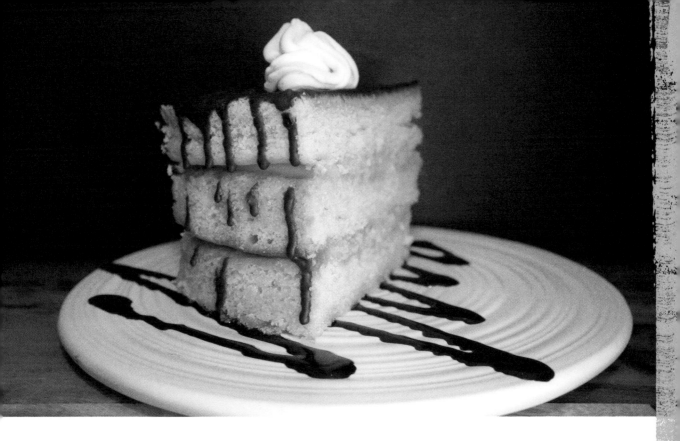

6   Add the flour mixture to the bowl with the wet ingredients. Whisk just until the batter is smooth and combined. Pour the batter into the prepared cake pans. Bake on the center rack until the tops are golden, the cakes pull away slightly from the sides of the pans, and a skewer inserted into the center of each cake comes out clean, 33 to 35 minutes. Let the cakes cool in the pans for 10 minutes, then invert them onto wire racks and let cool completely before filling.

7   Meanwhile, make the chocolate glaze: Put the chocolate chips in a deep heatproof bowl. In a small saucepan, combine the sugar and ¼ cup water. Bring to a boil over medium-high heat. Cook, stirring until the sugar has completely dissolved, about 2 minutes. Pour the sugar syrup over the chocolate, stir in the salt, and let stand, undisturbed, for 2 minutes.

8   Add the vanilla and brown rice syrup to the bowl with the chocolate and stir with a rubber spatula (do not use a whisk or it will create air bubbles) until the chocolate has melted and the glaze becomes glossy and smooth. Let stand for 5 minutes to thicken further.

9   Assemble the cake: Remove the parchment from the bottoms of the cake layers. Place one layer on a cake stand or plate. Spread half the vanilla custard over the top. Add another cake layer, then spread the remaining custard on top. Top with the remaining cake layer.

10 Spread the chocolate glaze over the top of the cake, letting it trickle down the sides, and serve.

TIP
Start the custard the night
before or early the morning
of, to avoid having to wait
for it to chill.

COCONUT CREAM PIE

SERVES 4   PREP TIME 20 MIN   CHILLING TIME 60 MIN   TOTAL TIME 1 HR 20 MIN

This raw, vegan, and gluten-free pie is so easy to prepare, it makes me wonder why I still eat processed foods. With about 20 minutes of prep and a few episodes of *The Office* while you're waiting for it to set in the fridge, you can have a whole coconut cream pie using fresh, simple ingredients! Peace Pies, located in sunny San Diego, doesn't cook any of their food past 105 degrees Fahrenheit. They use local ingredients and don't do much to alter the fruits, vegetables, nuts, and seeds. Their manager, Adam Miller, lost 160 pounds after his transition to a raw vegan diet. I was skeptical when he said he didn't have to sacrifice his sweet tooth to do it—until I tried their coconut cream pie. This dessert is refreshing and light, and the best part about it is that it uses only five ingredients. All you need other than those five ingredients are a food processor, a pie plate, and a fork. Enjoy!

1 cup hazelnuts

1 cup raisins

1/2 cup unsweetened shredded coconut

4 ripe bananas, peeled and broken into chunks

2 teaspoons cornstarch

Unsweetened cocoa powder, for dusting

Fresh strawberries, for serving

Store-bought chocolate sauce, for serving

1. Line an 8-inch pie plate with parchment paper (this will help the slices come out easier).

2. In a food processor, combine the hazelnuts and raisins. Pulse to break the nuts up a bit, then process until finely ground (the mixture will be sticky). Press the nut-raisin mixture evenly over the bottom and up the sides of the prepared pie pan.

3. Rinse and dry the food processor bowl and blade. Place the coconut, bananas, and cornstarch in the food processor. Pulse until smooth. Spoon the banana mixture over the crust and smooth it into an even layer. Refrigerate until firm enough to slice, at least 4 hours or up to overnight.

4. Dust with cocoa powder and serve with fresh strawberries and chocolate sauce.

From Trilogy Sanctuary in San Diego, California

GLUTEN-FREE CHOCOLATE BROWNIES

MAKES ONE 8-INCH TRAY   PREP TIME 10 MIN   COOKING TIME 20 TO 25 MIN
TOTAL TIME 30 TO 35 MIN

This recipe has to be one of the most memorable dishes I had on our *Evolving Vegan* tour for a few reasons. First of all, the actual space is stunning, and if you're ever in San Diego, you must visit Trilogy Sanctuary. Imagine an aerial yoga studio combined with a vegan, gluten-free, whole-food café all located on a vast rooftop that overlooks La Jolla, San Diego. Needless to say, not only was this one of the most peaceful places we visited on the tour, but this particular dish was the last of a vibrant, clean, healthy, delicious meal and took me by surprise. A warm, melt-in-your-mouth, gluten-free, soy-free vegan brownie topped with your choice of ice cream and a sweet chocolate sauce. Now *this* is a plant-based dessert you can feel good about indulging in and serving up to your friends!

1 tablespoon flaxseed meal

½ cup vegan chocolate chips (mini chips melt best, if you can find them)

¼ cup boiling water

⅓ cup coconut oil, warmed

1 teaspoon pure vanilla extract

¼ cup unsweetened cocoa powder

1 cup coconut sugar

¾ cup almond flour

1 teaspoon baking powder

Pinch of sea salt

Vegan coconut ice cream, for serving (optional)

1. Preheat the oven to 350°F. Line an 8-inch square baking dish with a piece of parchment paper, leaving a few inches overhanging the sides.

2. In a small bowl, whisk together the flaxseed meal and 2 tablespoons water. Let stand for 5 minutes; it will thicken to a soft, puddinglike consistency (this is called a "flax egg").

3. In a medium bowl, combine the chocolate chips, boiling water, and coconut oil. Let stand until the chocolate begins to melt, 1 to 2 minutes, then stir with a spatula until the chocolate is mostly melted. Stir in the vanilla.

4. In a medium bowl, whisk together the cocoa powder, sugar, almond flour, baking powder, and salt. Add the cocoa powder mixture and the flax egg to the melted chocolate mixture. Using a fork, stir just until there are no visible traces of the dry ingredients (the batter will be very thick).

5. Scrape the brownie batter into the prepared pan. Bake until firm and the top looks set, about 20 minutes. Let cool completely in the pan, then use the overhanging parchment to lift the brownies from the pan.

6. Serve warm, with vegan coconut ice cream, if you like.

TIP

Drizzle your favorite sauce over the brownie and sprinkle with crunchy cacao nibs.

ICE CREAM COOKIE SANDWICH

MAKES 1 QUART ICE CREAM AND 12 COOKIES
PREP TIME 30 MIN, PLUS AT LEAST 8 HRS CHILLING AND FREEZING
COOKING TIME 10 TO 12 MIN   TOTAL TIME 8 HRS 40 MIN

The chocolate chip cookie is a staple in every good cook's repertoire. But I thought it would be kind of boring if I just included a basic recipe. Here you not only get an all-around perfect cookie, but an ice cream to go between two of them. That's right—this is a chocolate chip cookie ice cream sandwich recipe! Now, I know not everyone is going to want to make ice cream from scratch, so if you don't have the time or inclination to, just make the cookies on their own—I promise they're amazing—and skip the ice cream part (or use store-bought vanilla ice cream instead). FoMu recommends you use 100% pure Madagascar vanilla extract and a real vanilla bean, but you can use Tahitian vanilla for a super-luxurious sweet treat as well. And for the ice cream, feel free to try almond extract instead of vanilla for a surprise twist. This recipe is completely plant-based and full of rich, sweet flavor. Real vanilla, a little coconut oil, and the sprinkling of some flaky sea salt are sure to make this one a staple in your recipe arsenal moving forward.

FOR THE VANILLA BEAN ICE CREAM

- 2 1/2 cups canned full-fat coconut milk
- 1/3 cup cane sugar
- 1/4 cup agave syrup
- 1 teaspoon pure vanilla extract
- 1 vanilla bean, split lengthwise and seeds scraped out

FOR THE CHOCOLATE CHIP COOKIES

- 1/2 cup vegan butter, at room temperature
- 2 tablespoons coconut oil
- 1/2 cup packed light brown sugar
- 1/2 cup cane sugar
- 1/4 cup unsweetened applesauce
- 1 teaspoon pure vanilla extract
- 2 1/2 cups all-purpose flour
- 3/4 teaspoon baking powder
- 1/2 teaspoon baking soda
- 1/2 teaspoon sea salt
- 1 cup dark chocolate chips
- Flaky sea salt, such as Maldon, for sprinkling

1   Make the vanilla bean ice cream: In a blender, combine the coconut milk, sugar, agave syrup, vanilla extract, and vanilla bean seeds. Blend until combined. Transfer to an airtight container and refrigerate for at least 4 hours or preferably overnight.

2   Pour the chilled mixture into an ice cream maker and churn according to the manufacturer's instructions. It should resemble soft-serve and hold to the scraper paddle when removed. Transfer to a freezer-safe container, tap the container against the counter to release any air bubbles, and freeze until the ice cream is firm enough to scoop, 4 to 6 hours.

3   Make the chocolate chip cookies: In a large bowl, combine the butter, coconut oil, and boths sugars and beat until creamy, 3 to 5 minutes. Add the applesauce and vanilla and beat until blended.

4   Add the flour, baking powder, baking soda, and salt and beat until just combined and there are no visible traces of flour. Stir in the chocolate chips. Cover the bowl with plastic wrap and refrigerate the dough for at least 30 minutes or up to overnight.

5   About 20 minutes before you're ready to bake the cookies, preheat the oven to 350°F. Line two rimmed baking sheets with parchment paper.

6   Drop 1/4- to 1/3-cup mounds of the dough onto the prepared baking sheets, spacing them at least 3 inches apart. Sprinkle the tops with a pinch of flaky salt.

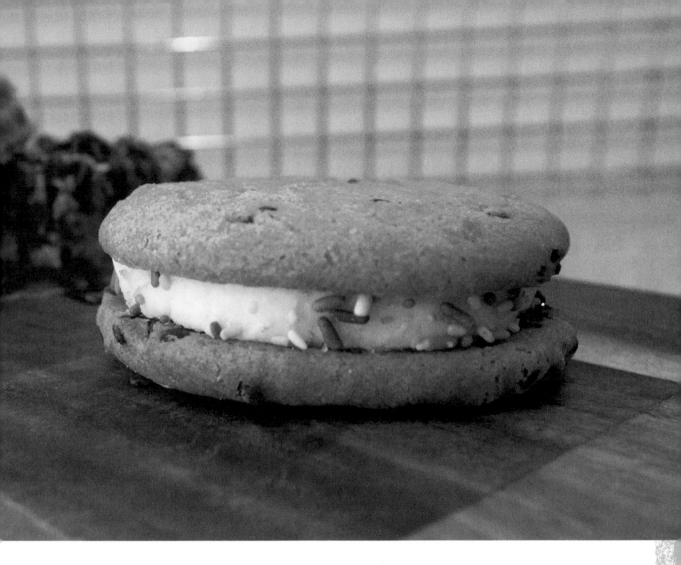

7 Bake the cookies until barely golden around the edges, 10 to 12 minutes. They will be very soft—let them cool on the baking sheet for 5 to 10 minutes before transferring them to a wire rack to cool completely.

8 Place a scoop of softened ice cream in the center of the flat side of one cooled cookie. Place a second cookie on top, flat side down, and gently press to form a sandwich.

TIPS

If you do not have an ice cream maker, feel free to use your favorite store-bought vanilla ice cream.

The cookies will keep in an airtight container at room temperature for up to 1 week or in the freezer for a couple of weeks.

Freezing your cookies before using them to make ice cream sandwiches will prevent breakage.

Freeze chunks of the dough for cookie dough ice cream or late-night nibbles!

CHOCOLATE MOUSSE WITH COCONUT DULCE DE LECHE

SERVES 6   **PREP TIME 30 MIN, PLUS 4 HRS CHILLING**   **COOKING TIME 2 HRS**
TOTAL TIME 6 HRS 30 MIN

Imagine a six-foot, bearded-and-tatted, *Sons of Anarchy*–looking man wearing an apron and delicately piping chocolate mousse onto a plate, then garnishing it with the most beautiful and aromatic mint leaf. That man is Chef Matthew Ravenscroft, in the beautiful kitchen at Rosalinda, located in the heart of one of the most popular cities in the world, Toronto. Chef Matt was kind enough to personally present and talk about each one of his dishes at this new, superbly popular vegan restaurant in Toronto. Mexico has long been known for its cultivation of cocoa plants, so it only makes sense that Chef Matt utilizes a beautiful dark chocolate to create this dish. I cannot explain to you how rich and flavorful this dessert is. It is so incredibly satisfying that once the mousse hits your palate, you will feel like you are standing in the middle of the most beautiful cocoa plantation in Tabasco, Mexico, while a mariachi band is singing at the top of their lungs and playing the *vihuela*. What I am trying to say is, if you like chocolate, make this now!

FOR THE CHOCOLATE MOUSSE

8 ounces dark or semisweet chocolate, finely chopped

16 ounces soft silken tofu

3 tablespoons pure maple syrup

2 tablespoons strong-brewed coffee, or 1 teaspoon instant espresso powder

¼ teaspoon sea salt

FOR THE DATE-CACAO CRUMBLE

1 ¼ cups unsweetened shredded coconut, toasted

½ cup dates, softened in hot water, thoroughly drained, and pitted

¼ cup unsweetened cocoa powder

¼ teaspoon sea salt

TO SERVE

¼ to ½ cup Coconut Milk Dulce de Leche (recipe follows)

Flaky sea salt, such as Maldon

1 to 1 ½ tablespoons buckwheat

Fresh mint leaves

TIP

Make sure you use silken tofu here or the mousse won't be smooth. You can make the mousse in advance so it chills properly.

1   Make the chocolate mousse: Fill a medium pot halfway with water and bring the water to a boil over high heat. Reduce the heat to maintain a vigorous simmer and place a heatproof bowl over the pot (it should be snug enough to act as a lid so there's no steam escaping; be sure the bottom of the bowl does not touch the water). Put the chocolate in the bowl and heat, stirring occasionally with a rubber spatula, until it has melted completely; remove the bowl from the pan and set aside to cool slightly. (Alternatively, you can put the chocolate in a microwave-safe bowl and microwave it in 30-second intervals, stirring after each, until completely melted.)

2   Meanwhile, in a blender, combine the tofu, maple syrup, coffee, and salt. Blend on high speed until completely pureed and smooth.

3   Add the melted chocolate to the blender and blend until fully combined and smooth, making sure there are no streaks of chocolate. Transfer the chocolate mousse to an airtight container, cover, and refrigerate until thoroughly chilled, at least 4 hours or up to overnight.

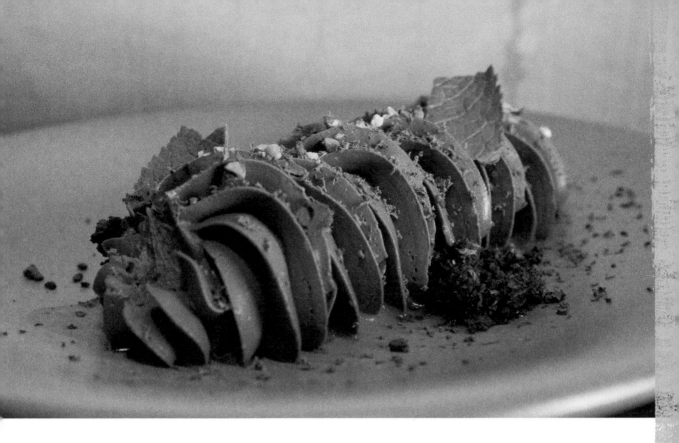

4   Next make the date-cacao crumble: In a food processor, combine the coconut, dates, cocoa powder, and salt and pulse until coarsely ground (the mixture will have a sticky, crumbly texture). Transfer to an airtight container and refrigerate until ready to use, up to 1 week.

5   When ready to serve, spoon the mousse into small serving bowls, or spoon it into a pastry bag fitted with a star tip and pipe it onto serving plates. Drizzle with some of the dulce de leche and sprinkle with a few flakes of sea salt, a few pieces of buckwheat, and some of the date-cocoa crumble. Garnish with mint leaves and serve.

COCONUT DULCE DE LECHE

(7.4-ounce) can sweetened condensed coconut milk

TIP
If your dulce de leche isn't as caramelized as you like, pour it into a small pot and cook over low heat, stirring frequently, until it reaches the desired color and consistency.

1   Remove the label from the can of condensed milk coconut but do not open the can. Place the can in a large pot and fill with enough water to cover the can by 4 inches, then bring to a boil.

2   Cook at a rolling boil for 2 hours, adding more water as needed to keep the can submerged by a few inches of water at all times, or else it will burst.

3   Using metal tongs, carefully remove the can from the water. Place it on a wire rack, unopened, and let cool completely.

4   Open the can, and you should have a golden-hued, caramel-like sauce. Use immediately or transfer to an airtight container and store in the refrigerator until ready to use, up to 3 days.

FRESH JAM WAFFLES

MAKES 4 TO 8 WAFFLES, DEPENDING ON THE SIZE OF YOUR WAFFLE IRON
PREP TIME 20 MIN   COOKING TIME 4 TO 5 MIN PER WAFFLE   TOTAL TIME 32 TO 40 MIN

I'm going to be honest about this recipe: If you don't have a waffle maker, just move on to the pancake recipe on page 28, because it's not going to be possible to make this. However, I wanted to include it in the book because whether you have kids you want to start a tradition with or it's your partner's birthday, homemade waffles always signify a special occasion. So it may be worth investing in a waffle maker just for this recipe, and to be honest, they're not that expensive anymore. Not to mention, this is a hearty, gluten-free waffle you can feel good about. The batter is always the hardest part, but the toppings are what make this dish your own and something you can have fun doing with your partner, kids, and loved ones.

2 ¼ cups gluten-free all-purpose flour

¼ cup buckwheat flour

2 tablespoons flaxseed meal

2 tablespoons cane sugar

1 tablespoon baking powder

½ teaspoon sea salt

2 cups unsweetened almond milk

¼ teaspoon pure vanilla extract

¼ cup neutral oil, such as grapeseed or safflower, or vegan butter, melted, plus more for coating

½ cup raspberry jam, warmed, for serving

½ cup orange marmalade, warmed, for serving

Mixed fresh berries, for serving

1   Preheat the oven to 300°F.

2   In a large bowl, whisk together the flours, flaxseed meal, sugar, baking powder, and salt.

3   Add the almond milk, vanilla, and oil and whisk to combine. Set the batter aside to rest for 10 minutes.

4   Meanwhile, preheat your waffle iron. Ladle some of the batter onto the waffle iron and cook according to the manufacturer's directions until golden brown and crispy. Transfer the waffle to a baking sheet; place the baking sheet in the oven to keep warm while you cook the remaining batter.

5   Serve the waffles with the warmed jam and marmalade and fresh berries on top.

TIP

These are also delicious plain or with vegan butter and maple syrup, avocado and fresh tomato salsa, or avocado and carrot "lox" (see page 19).

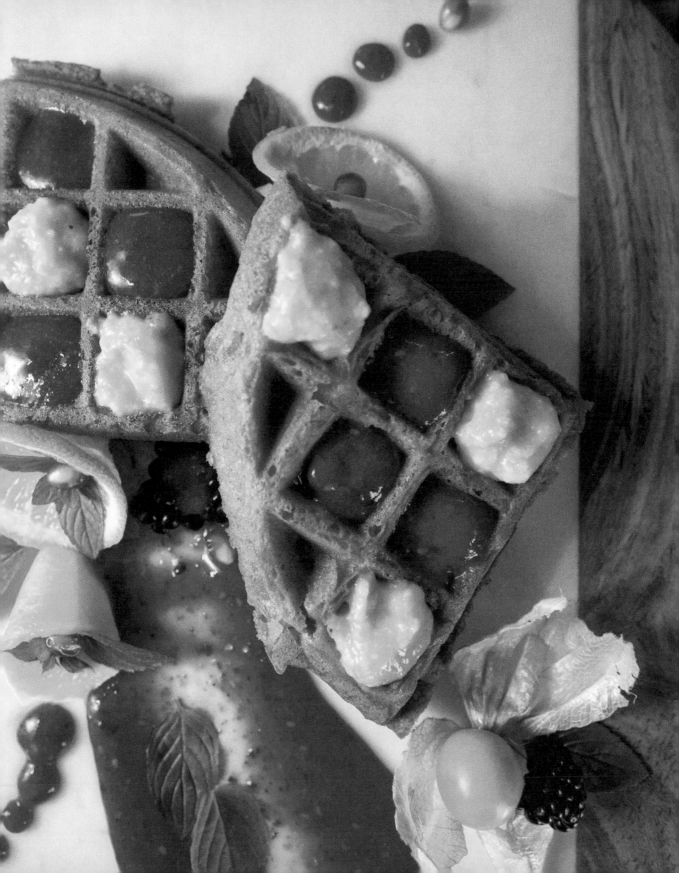

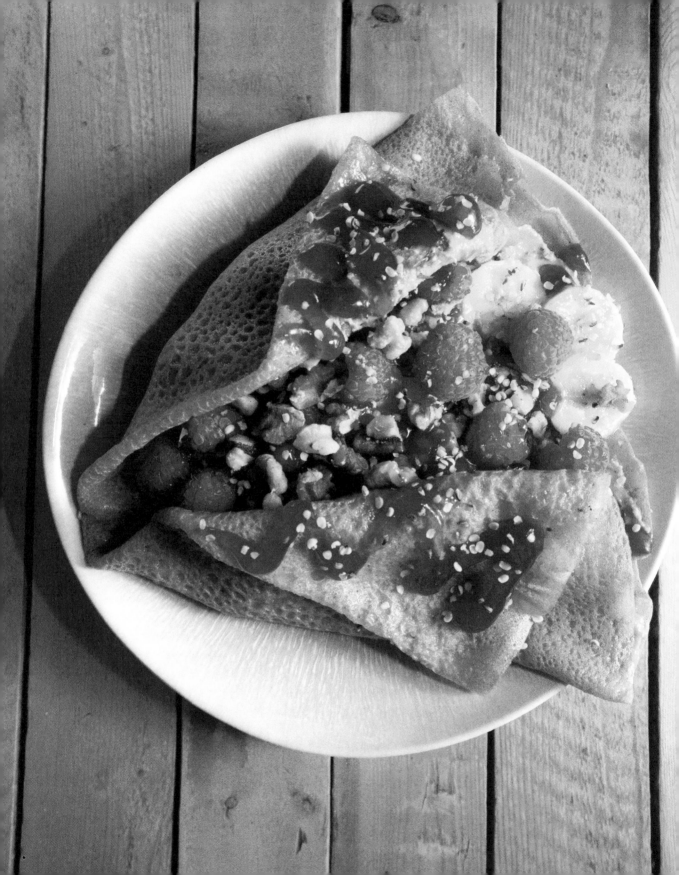

RAZZY RASBERRY CREPE

SERVES 6   PREP TIME 10 MIN   COOKING TIME 2 TO 4 MIN PER CREPE
TOTAL TIME 30 TO 40 MIN (INCLUDES 5 MIN RESTING TIME)

I don't know if I've ever met anyone who doesn't like raspberries. If you happen to be that one person, then substitute blueberries, or your favorite berries, every time you see "raspberry" in this recipe. Growing up, whenever my guy friends and I were feeling swanky (aka were in the company of girls), we would meet up at our local dessert shop. It was there that I cultivated my first relationships with . . . crepes. At first, I didn't really understand what a crepe was. It reminded me of that thin layer of egg left on your pan after you cooked an omelet; it was unappetizing, to say the least. But the more I had *good* crepes, the more I grew to love them, and this dessert crepe from Little Choc Apothecary in Brooklyn was the raspberry on top! This is light, fluffy, and so well balanced with raspberry jam, fresh raspberries, slices of banana, and crushed walnuts. Make sure to check out Little Choc the next time you're in Brooklyn, but until then, here's some razzy ras!

FOR THE BUCKWHEAT CREPES

1 ¼ cups nondairy milk of your choice (we used cashew)

¼ cup cornstarch

¼ cup buckwheat flour

½ cup gluten-free all-purpose flour

Pinch of sea salt

2 tablespoons vegan butter, melted

FOR THE FILLING

½ cup seedless raspberry jam

½ cup nut butter

½ pint fresh raspberries

1 banana, peeled and cut crosswise into ¼-inch-thick slices

½ cup walnuts, toasted and chopped

1 tablespoon hemp hearts

1   Make the crepes: Combine the milk, cornstarch, both flours, the salt, and butter in a blender. Blend until smooth and there are no visible lumps. Let the batter rest for 5 minutes, then pulse again once or twice just to recombine.

2   Heat an 8-inch nonstick skillet or crepe pan over medium heat. Pour in ¼ to ⅓ cup of the batter and swirl the skillet to completely coat the bottom in a thin layer of batter. Cook until the edges of the crepe appear dry and air bubbles form on top, 1 to 2 minutes, then flip the crepe and cook for 1 to 2 minutes more, until golden underneath and cooked through. Transfer to a plate, cover loosely with aluminum foil, and repeat to cook the rest of the batter.

3   When ready to serve, make the filling: Whisk the raspberry jam in a small bowl until smooth, adding water 1 teaspoon at a time, if necessary, to thin it slightly for drizzling. Spread some of the nut butter onto each crepe. Fold the crepe in half with the nut butter on the inside. Top with the raspberries, bananas, walnuts, and hemp hearts. Fold the outer edges of the crepe slightly over the filling. Drizzle with the raspberry jam and serve.

WASHIN DC

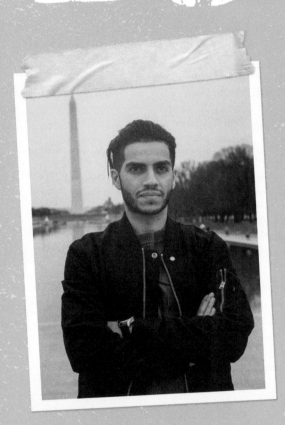

I HAVE A SPECIAL PLACE IN MY HEART FOR ANYTHING THAT IS AN "UNDERDOG," BECAUSE IT'S A TERM THAT I HAVE IDENTIFIED WITH MY WHOLE LIFE.

When my team made the case for Washington, DC, to be a part of our tour, I was a little dumbfounded. And because of that, it certainly was an underdog in my eyes, compared to all the other places we were visiting with unquestionable reputations for being exemplary vegan cities. I didn't expect much from the most political city in the world, but I have to say Washington vastly exceeded my expectations. It was home to some really interesting plant-based spots, including a bakery owned by a former *Cupcake Wars* champion, Doron Petersan, and the fanciest vegan fine-dining restaurant we visited on the tour, Elizabeth's Gone Raw, which is actually an old Victorian home turned restaurant. It's also the city where I discovered one of my personal favorite vegan

HERO SPOTLIGHT

DORON PETERSAN
Owner, Sticky Fingers and Fare Well

restaurants in North America: Fancy Radish. I expected nothing impressive from Washington, but I was blown away by what I found there.

The reason this boom of plant-based eateries is starting to happen in Washington is that the city has long been dominated by the baby boomers, but, like everywhere else in the world, younger generations are starting to take over, and with that comes a change in culture in everything from the arts scene to the culinary world. Spending time in Washington taught me that even the most unlikely places in the world are starting to evolve vegan. And with the most powerful fast-food chains starting to implement plant-based options, it's no surprise that even a city like Washington is starting to embrace the inevitable rise of plant-based lifestyles.

Chef Doron Petersan is in da houuussee! This enthusiasm is what I felt on the two occasions when I got to hang out with this amazing human being! With both a popular bakery and newly opened diner in Washington, DC, Doron is a busy boss woman! However, hanging out with her felt like spending time with one of my very best friends: she's easygoing, full of energy and spunk, and not to mention hilarious. Doron first knew she was onto something when her vegan cupcakes won her two titles on *Cupcake Wars*, making her a two-time champion. She's one of those vegans who adopted the lifestyle far before it was popular and opened her bakery in Washington in 2002. She's a great example of someone doing something they love and believe in, no matter what other people say. In fact, she recalls that during her time on *Cupcake Wars*, the term "vegan" was so foreign to viewers that she wasn't encouraged to call her cupcakes vegan or plant-based.

All this to say, Doron has endured many struggles to get to the point where she is now. And in a city where the adult population seems to be getting younger and younger and adapting more forward-thinking views, it's the perfect time to be Doron. Her bakery has almost twenty years of history and has become one of Washington's staples. On top of that, she has taken her experience and passion and opened up one of the hottest new restaurants in the city, Fare Well. There is no doubt in my mind her two creations will live on for another twenty years. So the next time you find yourself in Washington, DC, make sure to give my homie Chef Doron Petersan a shout!

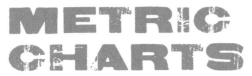

METRIC CHARTS

The recipes that appear in this cookbook use the standard US method for measuring liquid and dry or solid ingredients (teaspoons, tablespoons, and cups). The information on these pages is provided to help cooks outside the United States successfully use these recipes. All equivalents are approximate.

METRIC EQUIVALENTS FOR DIFFERENT TYPES OF INGREDIENTS

A standard cup measure of a dry or solid ingredient will vary in weight depending on the type of ingredient. A standard cup of liquid is the same volume for any type of liquid. Use the following chart when converting standard cup measures to grams (weight) or milliliters (volume).

STANDARD CUP	FINE POWDER (ex. flour)	GRAIN (ex. rice)	GRANULAR (ex. sugar)	LIQUID SOLIDS (ex. butter)	LIQUID (ex. milk)
1	140 g	150 g	190 g	200 g	240 ml
¾	105 g	113 g	143 g	150 g	180 ml
⅔	93 g	100 g	125 g	133 g	160 ml
½	70 g	75 g	95 g	100 g	120 ml
⅓	47 g	50 g	63 g	67 g	80 ml
¼	35 g	38 g	48 g	50 g	60 ml
⅛	18 g	19 g	24 g	25 g	30 ml

USEFUL EQUIVALENTS FOR DRY INGREDIENTS BY WEIGHT

(To convert ounces to grams, multiply the number of ounces by 30.)

OZ	LB	G
1 oz	¹/₁₆ lb	30 g
4 oz	¼ lb	120 g
8 oz	½ lb	240 g
12 oz	¾ lb	360 g
16 oz	1 lb	480 g

USEFUL EQUIVALENTS FOR LENGTH

(To convert inches to centimeters, multiply the number of inches by 2.5.)

IN	FT	YD	CM	M
1 in			2.5 cm	
6 in	½ ft		15 cm	
12 in	1 ft		30 cm	
36 in	3 ft	1 yd	90 cm	
40 in			100 cm	1 m

USEFUL EQUIVALENTS FOR LIQUID INGREDIENTS BY VOLUME

TSP	TBSP	CUPS	FL OZ	ML	L
¼ tsp				1 ml	
½ tsp				2 ml	
1 tsp				5 ml	
3 tsp	1 Tbsp		½ fl oz	15 ml	
	2 Tbsp	⅛ cup	1 fl oz	30 ml	
	4 Tbsp	¼ cup	2 fl oz	60 ml	
	5⅓ Tbsp	⅓ cup	3 fl oz	80 ml	
	8 Tbsp	½ cup	4 fl oz	120 ml	
	10⅔ Tbsp	⅔ cup	5 fl oz	160 ml	
	12 Tbsp	¾ cup	6 fl oz	180 ml	
	16 Tbsp	1 cup	8 fl oz	240 ml	
	1 pt	2 cups	16 fl oz	480 ml	
	1 qt	4 cups	32 fl oz	960 ml	
			33 fl oz	1000 ml	1 l

USEFUL EQUIVALENTS FOR COOKING/OVEN TEMPERATURES

	FAHRENHEIT	CELSIUS	GAS MARK
FREEZE WATER	32°F	0°C	
ROOM TEMPERATURE	68°F	20°C	
BOIL WATER	212°F	100°C	
	325°F	160°C	3
	350°F	180°C	4
	375°F	190°C	5
	400°F	200°C	6
	425°F	220°C	7
	450°F	230°C	8
BROIL			Grill

RESOURCES

The resources listed here are helpful tools for you to learn more about the food you put into your body. I did not include this section to sway you to go vegan. In fact, like most things in life, you may have a completely different takeaway than I did. The important thing is— it's *knowledge*. And knowledge is power.

LITERATURE

SALT, SUGAR, FAT
HOW THE FOOD GIANTS HOOKED US
BY MICHAEL MOSS

This book has nothing to do with veganism. It's just an incredibly insightful book about how addictive processed and packaged foods can really be, and how the United States has affected the whole world's food habits.

IN DEFENSE OF FOOD
AN EATER'S MANIFESTO
BY MICHAEL POLLAN

Michael Pollan is one of my favorite people writing about food, diet, and humans. He doesn't so much advocate for veganism as he does eating whole foods. And he always offers a unique way of thinking.

THE OMNIVORE'S DILEMMA
A NATURAL HISTORY OF FOUR MEALS
BY MICHAEL POLLAN

A lot of people may be confused as to why I included this book, as Pollan writes in it that if the whole world went vegan, it could actually lead to more complications within the food supply. My reasoning is, he's a thought-provoking writer and I want people to always see both sides.

SHOULD WE ALL BE VEGAN?
A PRIMER FOR THE 21ST CENTURY
BY MOLLY WATSON

This is a good "starter" book for anyone who wants to learn more about veganism. The author takes you through the evolution of veganism, covers celebrity vegans, and explores the challenges with going vegan. It really is a great book.

DOCUMENTARIES

COWSPIRACY: THE SUSTAINABILITY SECRET

This documentary was the cherry on top for me. It focuses on the effect of factory farming on the environment and our planet. This film was eye-opening for me and really inspired me to evolve vegan.

WHAT THE HEALTH

Not only focusing on diet, this very thought-provoking film also explores the impact of the pharmaceutical sector in our society. You may not agree with everything you see in this documentary, but it will certainly leave you thinking.

FOOD MATTERS

Nutrition, food, and health are the focus of this film. I always say the two main reasons I transitioned to a plant-based diet are the environment and my health, and this documentary really sheds a light on that.

THE GAME CHANGERS

This is a more recent documentary that highlights elite athletes who are plant-based. It debunks the myth that you have to eat animal products in order to compete at a high level as an athlete.

FOOD, INC.

This film often gets overlooked, but I like it because of its focus on factory farming and its effect on not only the environment and the animals but the employees who are hired to carry out this work.

EARTHLINGS

Warning: This documentary is incredibly graphic. Though it's not one of my favorites, it is one of the OGs. Released back in 2005, the film is narrated by Joaquin Phoenix, the man who recently won an Oscar for *Joker*. If you really want to see what's behind the curtain in factory farming, there's nothing quite like *Earthlings*.

Please remember, all these resources come with a bias. And it's important to try to understand both biases. In their simplest form, the biases will be: "Veganism is good for you and/or the planet" *or* "Veganism is not good for you and/or the planet." At the end of the day, the decision is yours to make. I know many people who are plant-based for two, three, ten years, and then revert back to being omnivores. There is no right or wrong answer. The reason I created Evolving Vegan is so we can all have a judgment-free conversation about this, or at least try to.

But I hope everyone would agree with this: We all need to start being very aware of what we put into our bodies, where it comes from, and how it affects our planet. We can no longer blindly consume what other people tell us to. We must question everything, and make an active decision while taking into consideration our health, the earth we live on, and the sources of our food.

ACKNOWLEDGMENTS

Thank you to my partners-in-crime, Amy and Cory, for agreeing to travel North America with me on a very humble budget to try to get this done. Your free-spirited nature inspires me to be less anal, quite frankly, and live life to the fullest. I need to try harder at that, I know! But you believed in me and the vision from the beginning, and for that, I will always be grateful.

My all-star team of creatives, Shelby Ito and Andrew "The Guac" Rowley: You stepped up to the plate and knocked out home runs every day. You were focused, driven, creative, and supportive, which is not easy to do. Ito, your laughter reminded me to stop stressing so much, and Rowley, our late-night bonding sessions back at the hotel kept me sane. What happens in North America, stays in North America.

Elma Begovic, thank you for joining us and extending a helping hand in whatever way we needed it that day! The hustle is real, and we needed you more than you know. Keep shining your light everywhere you go.

Anja, Matt, and everyone at Tiller Press. I will never take for granted those who believe in me and give me a chance! Even after all the incredible opportunities I've gotten in my life, it never escapes me just how hard it is to find people who truly believe in you. Thank you for being patient, guiding me, motivating me, and believing that a little Canadian kid who used to dress up as Peter Pan could fly around North America finding the best vegan eats on the continent!

My whole team at Folio Literary, Link, Viewpoint, AI— Samantha, Anthony, Sophie, Viet, and Derek. Especially you, Katherine—you have taught me so much about the literary world and guided me through the whole process. There were days my head was spinning, and you always had me trusting in the process! Brad, you work harder than anyone I know. I don't know what I would do without you, and I count my blessings every day that our paths crossed oh so many years ago. You encourage and motivate me to go after whatever it is I want, and I couldn't have done any of this without you!

Mamma, ohhhh! I wouldn't have had this deep love for food if it weren't for you. Your passion in the kitchen and the love you make your food with is unparalleled. Some of my fondest memories of growing up are of you in the kitchen, making ten, twelve dishes for Christmas dinner without breaking a sweat. You are an inspiration and a Michelin-star chef in my books. Thank you for sharing our family recipes with the world—I know they will love them as much as I do! More important, thank you for being the best mom a kid could ask for and making sure Margaret, Marian, and I were always fed and taken care of. It sounds simple, but I know how hard you worked and the sacrifices you had to make.

Dad, Margaret, and Marian, thanks for supporting Mom and me throughout this process—maybe contribute something next time, okay? I'm kidding. I love you.

Last but not least, thank you to all the inspiring, passionate, goofy, hardworking people who let me come into your restaurants and wreak havoc! Without you, I could not have done this. The plant-based community in every city I visited was truly inspiring. I am in awe of your compassion, talent, wisdom, and generosity, and I want you to know that you make up a cornerstone of each of your respective cities. The world is truly a better place because of you—thank you!

From the bottom of my heart, thank you to everyone who has picked up a copy of this book. Just by reading it and hopefully cooking some of these recipes and visiting some of these restaurants, you, too, have made a difference and contributed to a global effort to try to save the one thing that gives us life every day—our planet.

RESTAURANT INDEX

PLANTA YORKVILLE
Toronto, Canada
www.plantarestaurants.com

PURA VITA
Los Angeles, California
puravitalosangeles.com

RED LENTIL
Boston, Massachusetts
theredlentil.com

ROSALINDA
Toronto, Cananda
www.rosalindarestaurant.com

STICKY FINGERS SWEETS & EATS
Washington, DC
www.stickyfingersbakery.com

SWEET HART KITCHEN
Toronto, Canada
sweethartkitchen.com

TACO PARTY
Boston, Massachusetts
www.tacopartytruck.com

THE BUTCHER'S DAUGHTER
Los Angeles, California
www.thebutchersdaughter.com

THE BUTCHER'S SON
Oakland, California
www.thebutchersveganson.com

THE SUDRA
Portland, Oregon
www.thesudra.com

TRILOGY SANCTUARY
San Diego, California
www.trilogysanctuary.com

VEGGIE GALAXY
Cambridge, Massachusetts
www.veggiegalaxy.com

VIRTUOUS PIE
Vancouver, Canada
virtuouspie.com

WETHETRILLIONS
San Francisco, California
www.wethetrillions.com

YAMCHOPS
Toronto, Canada
yamchops.com

INDEX

Page numbers in *italics* refer to illustrations.

veganism, 8–11
    animals and, 9
    resources on, 178–79
Vinaigrette, Tahini, 75

Waffles, Fresh Jam, 170, *171*
wraps:
    Breakfast Wrap, 18
    Lettuce Wraps with Spicy Korean Brussels
        Sprouts & Tofu, 132–33, *133*
    Magical Mango Curry Wrap, 86–87, *87*
    Pineapple & Soy Curl Wraps, 50, *51*

Young Coconut Ceviche, 56, 57

zucchini:
    Giambotta Stew, 72, *73*
    Le Madrid Zucchini Noodles, *114*, 115

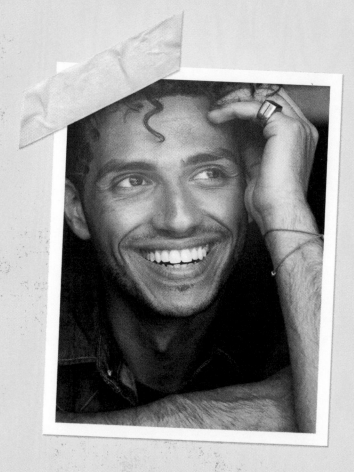

ABOUT THE AUTHOR

MENA MASSOUD was born in Cairo, Egypt. At the age of three, he immigrated to Toronto, Canada, with his parents and two sisters. He studied neuroscience at the University of Toronto and earned honor roll status before transferring to Ryerson University and graduating with a BFA in theatre. He is the founder of the company Evolving Vegan, which aims at making veganism accessible to all. Mena has also launched a nonprofit organization to aid underrepresented artists, the EDA (Ethnically Diverse Artists) Foundation, and a production company, Press Play Productions.

VANCOUVER

SEATTLE

PORTLAND

SAN FRANCISCO & OAKLAND

LOS ANGELES

SAN DIEGO